Hydrocephalus - Surgical Treatment

Edited by Amit Agrawal

Published in London, United Kingdom

Hydrocephalus - Surgical Treatment
http://dx.doi.org/10.5772/intechopen.1006398
Edited by Amit Agrawal

Contributors
Abed Alrazzak Kerhani, Alessandro Frati, Alexandru Vlad Ciurea, Aliyu Muhammad Koko, Amit Agrawal, Antonio Santoro, Deepal Attanayake, Giuseppa Zancana, Mattia Capobianco, Mauro Palmieri, Mohamed Yazbeck, Muhammad Mansur Idris, Nadun Danushka, Ravindri Jayasinghe, Valentin Titus Grigorean

Notice
Statements and opinions expressed in the chapters are these of the individual contributors and not necessarily those of the editors or publisher. No responsibility is accepted for the accuracy of information contained in the published chapters. The publisher assumes no responsibility for any damage or injury to persons or property arising out of the use of any materials, instructions, methods or ideas contained in the book.

First published in London, United Kingdom, 2025 by IntechOpen
IntechOpen is the global imprint of INTECHOPEN LIMITED, registered in England and Wales, registration number: 11086078, 167-169 Great Portland Street, London, W1W 5PF, United Kingdom

For EU product safety concerns: IN TECH d.o.o., Prolaz Marije Krucifikse Kozulić 3, 51000 Rijeka, Croatia, info@intechopen.com or visit our website at intechopen.com.

British Library Cataloguing-in-Publication Data
A catalogue record for this book is available from the British Library

Hydrocephalus - Surgical Treatment
Edited by Amit Agrawal
p. cm.
Print ISBN 978-1-83634-122-2
Online ISBN 978-1-83634-121-5
eBook (PDF) ISBN 978-1-83634-123-9

If disposing of this product, please recycle the paper responsibly.

IntechOpen

intechopen.com

Built by scientists, for scientists

Meet the editor

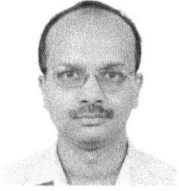

Dr. Agrawal completed his neurosurgery training at the National Institute of Mental Health and Neurosciences in Bangalore, India, in 2003. Dr Agrawal is a self-motivated, enthusiastic, and results-oriented professional with over 21 years of rich experience in research and development, as well as teaching and mentoring in the field of neurosurgery. He is proficient in managing and leading teams to run successful process operations and has experience in developing procedures and service standards of excellence. He has attended and participated in numerous international and national symposiums and conferences, delivering lectures on diverse topics. He has published over 1,000 articles in the medical field, covering a wide range of topics in national and international journals. His expertise lies in identifying training needs, designing training modules, and executing them while working with limited resources. He has excellent communication, presentation, and interpersonal skills with proven abilities in teaching and training for various academic and professional courses. Presently, he is working at the All-India Institute of Medical Sciences, Bhopal, Madhya Pradesh (India).

Contents

Preface

Hydrocephalus, characterized by the abnormal accumulation of cerebrospinal fluid (CSF) and the abnormal dilation of the brain's ventricles, may be caused by obstruction of the CSF pathways or, in some cases, by overproduction of the CSF. Despite significant advancements in diagnostics and treatment modalities, managing hydrocephalus remains complex and represents a multifaceted neurosurgical challenge across all age groups. The management of hydrocephalus requires careful clinical evaluation, precise clinical judgment, individualized interventional strategies, and follow-up.

The current book, *Hydrocephalus – Surgical Treatment*, considers all these details and brings together experienced contributors from various disciplines, including neurosurgeons, to present a comprehensive overview of current surgical approaches in the management of hydrocephalus. Subject experts share their clinical approach and surgical techniques, including pathophysiology, diagnosis, complications, and patient outcomes. The chapters cover a spectrum of clinical presentations ranging from normal pressure hydrocephalus to secondary causes, such as those arising from hemorrhage and trauma. The book emphasizes both conventional techniques, i.e., ventriculoperitoneal shunting.

Although this book provides a detailed review of surgical approaches to hydrocephalus, given the complexity of its etiology, presentation, and response to treatment, there will always be a need for high-quality, prospective, and randomized studies to inform evidence-based guidelines more effectively. We hope this volume will provide comprehensive reference material and a practical resource for neurosurgeons, neurologists, residents, and healthcare providers caring for patients with hydrocephalus. The current book aims to bridge clinical practice with research innovation, contributing meaningfully to the improvement of patient care and outcomes.

Amit Agrawal
Department of Neurosurgery,
All India Institute of Medical Sciences,
Saket Nagar, Bhopal, Madhya Pradesh, India

Chapter 1

Introductory Chapter: Hydrocephalus – Surgical Options

Amit Agrawal

1. Introduction

1.1 Hydrocephalus: Surgical options

Hydrocephalus is characterized by an abnormal accumulation of cerebrospinal fluid, which may or may not be associated with changes to intracranial pressure and varied clinical and radiological findings [1, 2]. It can be categorized into congenital or acquired based on etiology, communicating, or non-communicating based on the communication between the ventricular system and subarachnoid space through the foramen of Luschka and Magendie, or, less commonly, there may be overproduction of cerebrospinal fluid in the ventricular system [1, 3, 4]. Depending on the type of underlying etio-pathology, the site of cerebrospinal fluid (CSF) flow obstruction, the rapidity of onset, and the age of the patient (i.e., status of fontanelles open versus closed) clinical presentation shall vary [4, 5]. Acute presentation of hydrocephalus may include headache, impaired conscious level, vomiting, seizures, upward gaze paresis, diplopia, enlargement of the head in infants, and, less commonly, sudden death as in cases of colloid cyst of the third ventricle [5]. Normal Pressure Hydrocephalus (NPH) may present gait disturbances, urinary incontinence, and cognitive decline with or without headache [5]. The imaging work-up shall include ultrasonography in cases of neonates and infants, CT scan of the brain, and MRI of brain with flow studies (if needed) not only to diagnose but also to plan surgical versus conservative management strategy [5–10]. The understanding of the basic concepts is crucial to plan definitive management of hydrocephalus, particularly surgical options and approaches [1]. Once a diagnosis of symptomatic hydrocephalus is made, the surgical strategy may be directed toward removal of the obstruction of lesions compressing the CSF pathways of various CSF diversion procedures [11]. If needed in selected cases or in acute emergencies, the placement of temporary external drains may be considered [12]. The current work emphasizes on the ongoing advancements in the surgical management of hydrocephalus, correction selection of patients for surgical intervention, tailored surgical approaches, selection of catheters, minimally invasive procedures, immediate post-operative care, need for long-term follow-ups, and education and awareness of families to recognize features of shunt malfunctions and seek timely medical attention if there are symptoms of raised intracranial pressure [13, 14]. In the current volume experts share their views on third ventriculostomy in the context of ventriculoperitoneal shunt, alternative methods in the surgical treatment of hydrocephalus, the management of aqueductal stenosis, complications of ventriculoperitoneal shunt surgery, the role of endoscopic third ventriculostomy in the treatment of obstructive hydrocephalus, the management of idiopathic intracranial hypertension, and how to approach patients with post-traumatic hydrocephalus. While dealing with hydrocephalus it is a gentle reminder to consider other causes of large size and another controversial but important, that is, arrested hydrocephalus where there may be unique clinical presentations and management challenges [8, 15–20].

Author details

Amit Agrawal
Department of Neurosurgery, All India Institute of Medical Sciences, Bhopal, Madhya Pradesh, India

*Address all correspondence to: dramitagrawal@gmail.com; dramitagrawal@hotmail.com

IntechOpen

References

[1] Hochstetler A, Raskin J, Blazer-Yost BL. Hydrocephalus: Historical analysis and considerations for treatment. European Journal of Medical Research. 2022;**27**(1):168

[2] Mokri B. The Monro-Kellie hypothesis: Applications in CSF volume depletion. Neurology. 2001;**56**(12):1746-1748

[3] Ramesh VG, Narasimhan V, Balasubramanian C. Cerebrospinal fluid dynamics study in communicating hydrocephalus. Asian Journal of Neurosurgery. 2017;**12**(2):153-158

[4] Amen MM, Badran M, Zaher A, Khalil AF, Abdelaal I, Saad M. The outcome of surgical management of post-infectious hydrocephalus with multiple intraventricular septations. Egyptian Journal of Neurosurgery. 2023;**38**(1):65

[5] Krovvidi H, Flint G, Williams AV. Perioperative management of hydrocephalus. BJA Education. 2018;**18**(5):140-146

[6] McAuley D, Paterson A, Sweeney L. Optic nerve sheath ultrasound in the assessment of paediatric hydrocephalus. Child's Nervous System. 2009;**25**(1):87-90

[7] Singhal A, Yang MMH, Sargent MA, Cochrane DD. Does optic nerve sheath diameter on MRI decrease with clinically improved pediatric hydrocephalus? Child's Nervous System. 2013;**29**(2):269-274

[8] Panigrahi MK, Kodali S, Chandrsekhar Y, Vooturi S. Diagnostic nuances and surgical management of arrested hydrocephalus. Neurology India. 2021;**69**(Suppl.):S336-Ss41

[9] Pindrik J, Schulz L, Drapeau A. Diagnosis and surgical management of neonatal hydrocephalus. Seminars in Pediatric Neurology. 2022;**42**:100969

[10] Rich P, Jones R, Britton J, Foote S, Thilaganathan B. MRI of the foetal brain. Clinical Radiology. 2007;**62**(4):303-313

[11] Bergsneider M, Miller C, Vespa PM, Hu X. Surgical management of adult hydrocephalus. Neurosurgery. 2008;**62**(Suppl. 2):643-659; discussion 59-60

[12] Park EK, Kim JY, Kim DS, Shim KW. Temporary surgical management of intraventricular hemorrhage in premature infants. Journal of Korean Neurosurgical Association. 2023;**66**(3):274-280

[13] Zielińska D, Rajtar-Zembaty A, Starowicz-Filip A. Cognitive disorders in children's hydrocephalus. Neurologia i Neurochirurgia Polska. 2017;**51**(3):234-239

[14] Saad M, Raafat M, Zaher A, Badr H. Ventricular shunting paradigm in surgical management of arrested hydrocephalus in children with distorted mental status. The Medical Journal of Cairo University. 2019;**87**(12):5263-5268

[15] Hong J, Barrena BG, Lollis SS, Bauer DF. Surgical management of arrested hydrocephalus: Case report, literature review, and 18-month follow-up. Clinical Neurology and Neurosurgery. 2016;**151**:79-85

[16] Fukuhara T, Luciano MG. Clinical features of late-onset idiopathic aqueductal stenosis. Surgical Neurology. 2001;**55**(3):132-136; discussion 6-7

[17] Larsson A, Stephensen H, Wikkelsø C. Adult patients with "asymptomatic" and "compensated" hydrocephalus benefit from surgery. Acta Neurologica Scandinavica. 1999;**99**(2):81-90

[18] Locatelli M, Draghi R, Di Cristofori A, Carrabba G, Zavanone M, Pluderi M, et al. Third ventriculostomy in late-onset idiopathic aqueductal stenosis treatment: A focus on clinical presentation and radiological diagnosis. Neurologia Medico-Chirurgica (Tokyo). 2014;**54**(12):1014-1021

[19] Schick RW, Matson DD. What is arrested hydrocephalus? The Journal of Pediatrics. 1961;**58**:791-799

[20] Torkelson RD, Leibrock LG, Gustavson JL, Sundell RR. Neurological and neuropsychological effects of cerebral spinal fluid shunting in children with assumed arrested ("normal pressure") hydrocephalus. Journal of Neurology, Neurosurgery, and Psychiatry. 1985;**48**(8):799-806

Chapter 2

Aqueductal Stenosis: Pathophysiology, Diagnosis, and Treatment Modalities

Mohamed Yazbeck and Abed Alrazzak Kerhani

Abstract

Aqueductal stenosis is the primary cause of congenital and acquired hydrocephalus, which results from an obstruction in cerebrospinal fluid (CSF) flow through the cerebral aqueduct. The condition causes increasing intracranial pressure and progressive ventricular dilution that requires acute surgical intervention. Two of the primary treatment choices are ventriculoperitoneal (VP) shunting and endoscopic third ventriculostomy (ETV). Although VP shunting is still quite common, it has long-term side effects including shunt dependency, malfunction, and infection. By restoring CSF circulation, ETV presents a physiological substitute; yet, success rates depend on patient age, etiology, and anatomical factors. Rising approaches are ETV with choroid plexus cauterization, neuronavigation-assisted surgeries, and robotic-assisted neuroendoscopy, which is improving surgical results. Despite these advances, there nevertheless remain challenges in optimizing patient selection and minimizing postoperative complications. Emphasizing clinical decision-making and long-term management, this review offers an in-depth examination of the pathophysiology, diagnostic tools, and transforming surgical approaches for aqueductal stenosis.

Keywords: Aqueductal stenosis, hydrocephalus, endoscopic third ventriculostomy, ventriculoperitoneal shunting, cerebrospinal fluid dynamics, neurosurgical interventions, minimally invasive neurosurgery

1. Introduction

A well-known cause of congenital hydrocephalus, aqueductal stenosis accounts for either 6–66% of cases in children and 5–49% in adults [1]. It arises from a constriction or occlusion of the cerebral aqueduct (aqueduct of Sylvius), the narrowest segment of the cerebrospinal fluid (CSF) channel linking the third and fourth ventricles. This disorder causes the lateral and third ventricles to dilate while the fourth ventricle stays normal in size—a characteristic distinctive on neuroimaging [2]. Prenatally, usually as early as the midtrimester ultrasound scan, congenital aqueductal stenosis can be found and has important clinical consequences including neurodevelopmental delay, seizures, and early surgical intervention needed [3]. Considered to be 1 in 1000 live births, congenital hydrocephalus is thought to be caused mostly by aqueductal stenosis [3].

IntechOpen

Over time, the treatment of aqueductal stenosis has changed mostly to include endoscopic third ventriculostomy (ETV) and ventriculo-peritoneal (VP) shunting. First presented in the 1950s, the VP shunt is still a commonly performed operation because of its technical simplicity and somewhat low perioperative mortality (0.1–0.13%) when compared to ETV (1–10%). Long-term problems include infection, malfunction, and over-drainage, however call for regular changes; shunt failure rates within 2 years [2] approach 50%. On the other hand, ETV has become somewhat well-known as a physiological method avoiding foreign body implantation and preserving more natural CSF dynamics, especially since the 1990s [1]. Notwithstanding its benefits, ETV is a technically difficult operation with a large learning curve; its success rates rely on patient age, past infections, and the presence of other diseases [2]. Although a lot of research exists comparing the effectiveness of various therapies, a clear agreement is still difficult because of variability in study populations, follow-up times, and different definitions of treatment success [2]. Moreover, unresolved issues about the long-term neurodevelopmental issues in newborns treated with ETV along with the clinical relevance of ongoing ventriculomegaly following effective diversion surgeries [1] still remain.

This chapter is based on several studies, including a full overview of the current research on the surgical treatment of aqueductal stenosis, therefore providing an entire and well-rounded controversy. Carefully selecting studies based on their relevance, design, and quality of evidence, we analyzed peer-reviewed journal articles, systematic reviews, and meta-analyses from reputable databases involving PubMed, Scopus, and Web of Science. Clinical trials, retrospective analyses, and large-scale cohort studies comparing ETV and VP shunting took priority for an objective assessment of therapy efficacy.

Beyond published studies, we also included data from neurosurgery textbooks, reference books, and clinical guidelines from credible neurosurgical and pediatric resources. Regarding surgical procedures, patient selection, and long-term outcomes, these sources helped in shaping consensus recommendations and best practices. Moreover, we compiled statistical data on surgical success rates, complication risks, and long-term prognosis in order to provide a data-driven perceptions of treatment decisions.

Apart from going over the findings of recent studies, this chapter combines situations from our own clinical experience to present practical real-world guidance on managing aqueductal stenosis. These cases show the nuances of surgical decision-making, the difficulties encountered during these operations, and the corresponding postoperative outcomes. This combination of recent research with hands-on experience aimed to present a balanced, up-to-date, and clinically relevant discussion on the surgical management of aqueductal stenosis.

This chapter will give a full overview of the surgical treatment options for aqueductal stenosis, with an emphasis on their indications, procedures, and results.

2. Anatomy and surgical considerations of the cerebral aqueduct

Comprising a network of connected cavities in the brain, the ventricular system contains cerebrospinal fluid (CSF). Protection of the brain, maintenance of intracraneural pressure, and CSF circulation depend on it. Connected by specialized pathways regulating cerebrospinal fluid flow, the system consists of four main ventricles: the paired lateral ventricles, the third ventricle, and the fourth ventricle [4].

The lateral ventricles are nestled within each cerebral hemisphere, making them the largest and most crucial component of the ventricular system. They are made up of an anterior (frontal), a body, a posterior (occipital), and an inferior (temporal) horn. Via the foramina of Monro, sometimes known as interventricular foramina, these ventricles connect to the third ventricle. Bordered by the thalamus and hypothalamus, the third ventricle is a narrow, slit-like cavity found midway between the two halves of the diencephalon [5]. The third ventricle, a thin passage within the midbrain, descends and connects to the fourth ventricle via the cerebral aqueduct. This fourth ventricle lies between the brainstem and the cerebellum and the subarachnoid space, consisting of the terminal ventricular cavity before cerebrospinal fluid enters the spinal cord's central canal. Through the median aperture (foramen of Magendie) and the lateral apertures (foramina of Luschka), the fourth ventricle connects to the subarachnoid space, enabling the flow of cerebrospinal fluid around the brain and spinal cord [6].

Figure 1 provides a detailed left lateral view of the human ventricular system, illustrating the spatial orientation of the ventricles and their connections. This anatomical representation enhances the understanding of CSF dynamics and the potential sites of obstruction that can contribute to conditions such as hydrocephalus.

2.1 The cerebral aqueduct and its role in CSF flow

2.1.1 Relevance to the anatomical structures

The cerebral aqueduct, also known as the aqueduct of Sylvius, is a narrow tubular structure located in the midbrain, with a diameter of 1–2 mm. It functions as the exclusive conduit for cerebrospinal fluid (CSF) movement between the third and fourth ventricles. This particular anatomical orientation allows for the control of intracranial pressure (ICP) and cerebrospinal fluid (CSF) circulation. Whether congenital, neoplastic, post-hemorrhagic, or inflammatory, disruptions in aqueductal patency cause proximal cerebrospinal fluid accumulation, resulting in ventriculomegaly and elevated intracranial pressure—features of obstructive hydrocephalus [6].

The cerebral aqueduct holds strategic significance in cerebrospinal fluid physiology due to its role as a bottleneck in the ventricular system. In contrast to the foramina

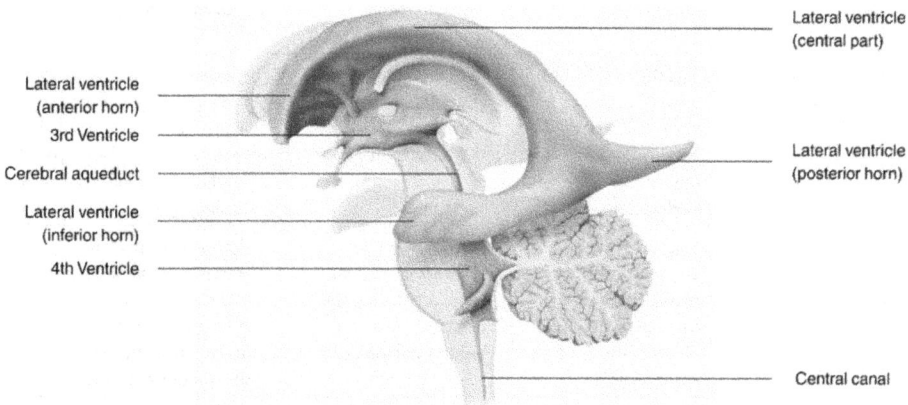

Figure 1.
Human ventricular system (left lateral view).

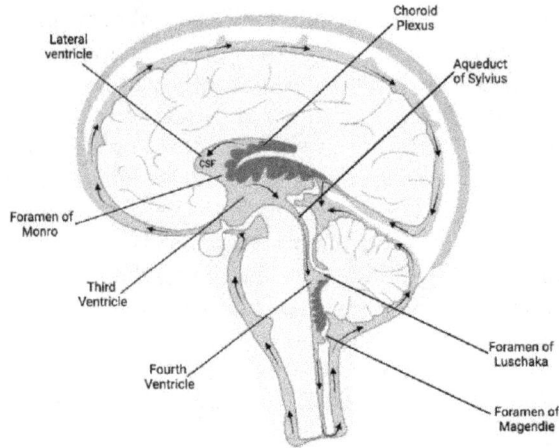

Figure 2.
Ventricular system—pathway of cerebrospinal fluid flow. Source: Byron et al. [8]. Licensed under CC BY 4.0.

Anatomical structure	Surgical challenge	Potential complications	Mitigation strategies
Basilar Artery (BA) and perforators	Located ventral to the third ventricle floor, making them susceptible to injury during procedures like endoscopic third ventriculostomy (ETV).	Injury can lead to brainstem ischemia, pontine infarcts, oculomotor palsy, or catastrophic hemorrhage.	Utilize preoperative imaging to assess vascular proximity, plan precise endoscopic trajectories, and employ gentle perforation techniques to minimize risk [7].
Foramen of Monro	May be narrow or obstructed due to congenital anomalies, tumors, or adhesions, complicating endoscopic access.	Restricted instrument maneuverability can result in forniceal injury, leading to memory impairment.	Use neuronavigation to guide approach, consider staged dilation or septostomy to improve access, and monitor for signs of forniceal injury [9].
Mammillary bodies and hypothalamus	Located near standard ETV perforation sites, increasing risk of inadvertent damage during surgery.	Damage can cause anterograde amnesia, hypothalamic dysfunction, or Korsakoff-like symptoms.	Identify anatomical landmarks preoperatively, exercise caution with endoscopic instruments, and avoid excessive manipulation near these structures [7].
Variability in third ventricle floor morphology	The floor's thickness and transparency vary; thicker or opaque floors present higher resistance to perforation.	Incomplete ETV, need for repeat surgery, or increased risk of vascular injury.	Assess floor characteristics intraoperatively, use appropriate instruments for controlled perforation, and be prepared to adjust techniques based on findings [7].
Liliequist membrane and secondary obstructions	Failure to recognize and perforate this membrane can cause persistent CSF obstruction despite a successful ETV.	Incomplete CSF diversion, ongoing hydrocephalus, and potential need for additional interventions.	Routinely inspect the interpeduncular cistern intraoperatively, confirm free CSF flow before concluding surgery, and address any secondary obstructions as needed [7].

Table 1.
Anatomical challenges, complications, and mitigation strategies in endoscopic third ventriculostomy (ETV) for aqueductal stenosis.

of Monro or the foramina of Luschka and Magendie, which offer alternative pathways for cerebrospinal fluid (CSF), the aqueduct does not possess collateral routes. Consequently, even minor obstructions can have significant implications [7].

Figure 2 shows the ventricular system and the path of cerebrospinal fluid flow, emphasizing the role of the aqueduct as the main conduit between the supratentorial and infratentorial compartments.

2.2 Anatomical challenges for surgeons

2.2.1 Proximity to vital structures and implications for surgical planning

Deep location and proximity to important neurovascular structures make surgical interventions that involve the cerebral aqueduct and third ventricle challenging. Minimizing risks and enhancing patient outcomes depend on the understanding of these anatomical relationships.

Key anatomical structures, associated surgical challenges possible complications, and techniques to reduce these risks are summarized in the following **Table 1**.

Successful surgical results in operations involving the cerebral aqueduct and third ventricle depend on understanding these anatomical difficulties and application of suitable techniques [10].

3. Pathophysiology of aqueductal stenosis and indications for surgery

3.1 Mechanisms of obstruction

3.1.1 Congenital causes of aqueductal stenosis

3.1.1.1 Embryological development and anatomic considerations

Early embryonic development produces the cerebral aqueduct as a small channel inside the mesencephalon. Originally the same size as other parts of the ventricular system, the lumen of the aqueduct narrows gradually as a result of the thickening of surrounding neural structures, including the superior and inferior colliculi [1]. The aqueduct's natural narrowing renders it easily blocked in pathological conditions.

Four primary types [1] have been established by histopathological studies for congenital aqueductal stenosis:

- Simple stenosis: Constriction of the aqueduct characterized by ependymal cell lining and the absence of gliosis. Atypical neural tube infolding during development might be the cause.

- Forking: The aqueduct is split into multiple channels, some of which might close abruptly, therefore disrupting the usual flow of cerebrospinal fluid (CSF).

- Septal formation: Usually from constant pressure and canal stretching, which closes the glial membrane and blocks the aqueduct.

- Gliotic stenosis: Reactive gliosis and glial overgrowth replace the normal ependymal lining, therefore blocking the lumen and CSF flow.

Hydrocephalus – Surgical Treatment

Characterized by mutations in the L1CAM gene [1], congenital anomalies can be idiopathic or associated with genetic disorders, including X-linked hydrocephalus (L1 syndrome) (**Figure 3**).

3.1.1.2 Genetic factors

Aqueductal stenosis can arise from gene alterations associated with cell adhesion and neural tube formation. The most widely investigated genetic condition associated with congenital aqueductal stenosis is X-linked hydrocephalus (L1 syndrome). Mutations in the L1CAM gene—which codes for a neural cell adhesion molecule essential for neuronal migration and axon development [12]—cause this disorder. Aqueductal stenosis is often the result of chronic compression caused by the expansion of the lateral and third ventricles.

Usually occurring alongside optic pathway gliomas, congenital disorders related to aqueductal stenosis include neurofibromatosis type 1 in about 5% of individuals [1].

The downward displacement of the cerebellar tonsils and brainstem in Chiari malformation type II may cause compression of the aqueduct [1].

Dandy-Walker malformation, along with an enlarged fourth ventricle and a hypoplastic or dysplastic cerebellum, can cause aqueductal obstruction [1].

3.1.2 Acquired causes of aqueductal stenosis

3.1.2.1 Post-Hemorrhagic and post-infectious stenosis

Intraventricular hemorrhage (IVH) is a leading cause of acquired aqueductal stenosis, particularly in preterm neonates. Formation of clots and later fibrosis can obstruct the aqueduct, causing hydrocephalus [1]. The gliotic response to IVH might cause the aqueduct to gradually narrow and obliterate completely.

Likewise, infectious agents including bacterial meningitis or viral encephalitis—such as cytomegalovirus, mumps, and lymphocytic choriomeningitis virus—can

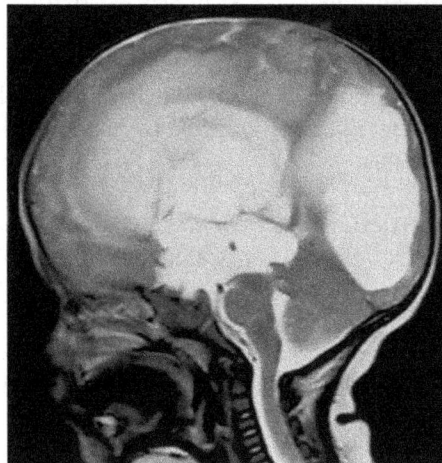

Figure 3.
An ideal candidate for ETV at six and half months of age due to congenital aqueduct stenosis with dilated third ventricle, floor bulging down into the interpeduncular cistern and adequate pre-pontine space. Source: Deopujari et al. [11]. Licensed under CC BY 3.0.

10

cause ependymal inflammation, which results in gliosis and subsequently stenosis [1]. In these situations, scarring may develop gradually, or inflammatory debris may lead to acute CSF flow restriction.

3.1.2.2 Disruption of ventricular zone integrity

The ventricular zone (VZ) consists of radial glia/neural stem cells responsible for neurogenesis. Whether via genetic defects or secondary injuries, disturbance of this area might hinder the development of normal CSF routes. Studies in hydrocephalic mouse models—e.g., the hyh mutant mouse—have shown that aberrant cell connections and ependymal cell loss in the Sylvian aqueduct (SA) precede aqueductal stenosis [12].

Key cellular alterations causing aqueductal stenosis include:

- Reduced ependymal cell density brought on by poor cell adhesion and elevated death rate.

- Development of subependymal glial scarring, gradually narrowing the aqueduct.

- Abnormal localization of N-cadherin and connexin 43, disrupting the adherens and gap junctions required for ventricular zone integrity [12].

3.1.2.3 Trauma and tumors

Tectal gliomas, pineal area tumors, ependymomas, and space-occupying lesions in the posterior fossa can compress the aqueduct externally, causing an occlusion. Traumatic brain injury can also cause ventricular distortion, thus narrowing the aqueduct (**Table 2**) [1].

In neurosurgery, aqueductal stenosis remains a major pathology that calls for precise diagnostic imaging and personalized surgical intervention. Understanding the mechanisms of both acquired and congenital types of stenosis guides choices for treatment and current hydrocephalus management studies.

Cause	Pathophysiological mechanism	Examples
Congenital malformations	Developmental errors leading to narrowed or divided aqueduct	X-linked hydrocephalus, Chiari II, Dandy-Walker
Genetic defects	Mutations affecting cell adhesion and neurogenesis	L1CAM mutation, neurofibromatosis type 1
Post-hemorrhagic	Clot formation, fibrosis, and gliosis	Preterm IVH, ruptured aneurysm
Post-infectious	Inflammation and ependymal damage leading to stenosis	CMV, mumps, bacterial meningitis
Ventricular zone disruption	Loss of ependymal integrity, gliosis, and stenosis	Hyh mouse model, connexin/N-cadherin defects
External compression	Mass effect from tumors or posterior fossa anomalies	Tectal glioma, pineal tumors

Table 2.
Etiologies and mechanisms of aqueductal stenosis.

3.2 Impact of stenosis on CSF dynamics: Ventricular dilation and intracranial pressure

Aqueductal stenosis seriously impacts cerebrospinal fluid (CSF) dynamics, causing increasing intracranial pressure (ICP) and gradual ventricular dilatation. Normal CSF flow from the third to the fourth ventricle is blocked at the cerebral aqueduct, leading to a buildup of CSF in the lateral and third ventricles while the fourth ventricle remains unaffected [13]. Reduced cerebral compliance, mechanical compression of periventricular structures, and shifted cerebral perfusion follow this disturbance and contribute to neurological deterioration.

3.2.1 Ventricular dilation and structural changes

3.2.1.1 Pathophysiology of ventricular enlargement

Aqueductal stenosis results in triventricular hydrocephalus, characterized by a disproportionate dilation of the lateral and third ventricles while sparing the fourth ventricle [13]. The main mechanisms include the following:

- Increased intraventricular pressure gradient: Due to restricted outflow, along with the continued production of CSF at a normal rate (~500 mL/day), CSF accumulates in the upstream ventricles, causing progressive expansion [13].

- Periventricular ischemia: In chronic cases [13], the continuous pressure on the ependymal lining distorts CSF absorption, leading to periventricular edema, neuronal loss, and up to a 40% decrease in periventricular white matter volume.

- Disturbance in periventricular structures: Mechanical stretching of the corpus callosum and fornices causes memory problems in 40% of individuals with chronic hydrocephalus [14].

3.2.1.2 Imaging markers of ventricular dilation

Objective evidence of ventricular dilatation provided by MRI and CT scan include:

- Increase in ventricular index: Lateral and third ventricle enlargement by 30–50% relative to normal controls [14].

- Periventricular edema: Indicates trans-ependymal CSF absorption and persistent pressure overload. Seen in 60–75% of symptomatic patients [13].

- Third ventricle ballooning: Occurs in up to 25% of cases [13], causing compression of the pituitary stalk and hypothalamus, thereby affecting the endocrine system.

- Evans's Index (EI) > 0.3: Found in over 90% of diagnosed cases [14], this is a crucial diagnostic marker of ventricular enlargement.

3.2.2 Intracranial pressure alterations in Aqueductal stenosis

3.2.2.1 Physiological changes in ICP

CSF pressure dynamics in aqueductal stenosis are characterized by the following:

- Increased opening pressure on lumbar puncture (mean 13.95 ± 2.88 mmHg, with peaks surpassing 20 mmHg in acute cases) [14].

- Impaired CSF absorption and higher pressure gradients, demonstrated by elevated resistance to outflow (Rout ~11.21 ± 2.00 mmHg/mL/min) [14].

- ICP waveform abnormalities, including plateau waves and decreased intracranial compliance, found in 50–60% of individuals undergoing continuous ICP monitoring [14] .

- Reduced cerebral compliance, which raises ICP variations in response to small volume changes; compliance indices show a 30% drop from healthy people [14].

3.2.2.2 Clinical consequences of ICP elevation

In untreated aqueductal stenosis, continuous ICP increase produces the following:

- Headache and nausea, noted in 80% of symptomatic patients [14], intensify in the morning due to temporary ICP increases during sleep.

- Papilledema, an indication of ongoing intracranial hypertension, is observed in 35–50% of cases [13].

- Cognitive impairment, affecting more than 40% of individuals with chronic hydrocephalus [14], is mostly associated with memory problems caused by compression of periventricular structures.

- Acute herniation, which occurs in 10–15% of emergency patients and requires immediate decompression via surgery.

3.2.3 CSF flow disruptions and post-treatment effects

3.2.3.1 Pre- and post-operative CSF flow findings

Phase-contrast MRI and cine MRI CSF flow studies show notable changes both before and after endoscopic third ventriculostomy (ETV):

- Pre-operative: Absence of aqueductal flow void, turbulent CSF motion in the third ventricle, and significant periventricular edema—observed in 80–90% of untreated cases [13].

- Post-operative: With 75–85% of patients experiencing considerable clinical improvement, these changes include restoration of pulsatile CSF flow through the third ventricle floor, reduced ventricular size, and normalizing of periventricular perfusion (**Figure 4**) [13].

The primary cause of ventricular enlargement and increased ICP is aqueductal stenosis-induced CSF flow disturbance, necessitating timely intervention to prevent permanent neurological damage. With reported success rates of 70–90% depending on patient age and etiology [13, 14], ETV remains the preferred treatment, effectively restoring CSF dynamics while reducing long-term shunt dependency.

3.3 Indications for surgical intervention: Symptomatic hydrocephalus, refractory cases, and risk of acute decompensation

Surgical intervention in aqueductal stenosis is primarily indicated for patients with symptomatic hydrocephalus, those who have not responded to initial treatment, and individuals at risk of sudden neurological deterioration. Clinical symptoms, imaging findings, and disease progression guide surgical decisions [16, 17].

3.3.1 Symptomatic hydrocephalus

Patients with symptomatic hydrocephalus often experience papilledema, nausea, vomiting, and headaches due to elevated intracranial pressure (ICP). Studies indicate

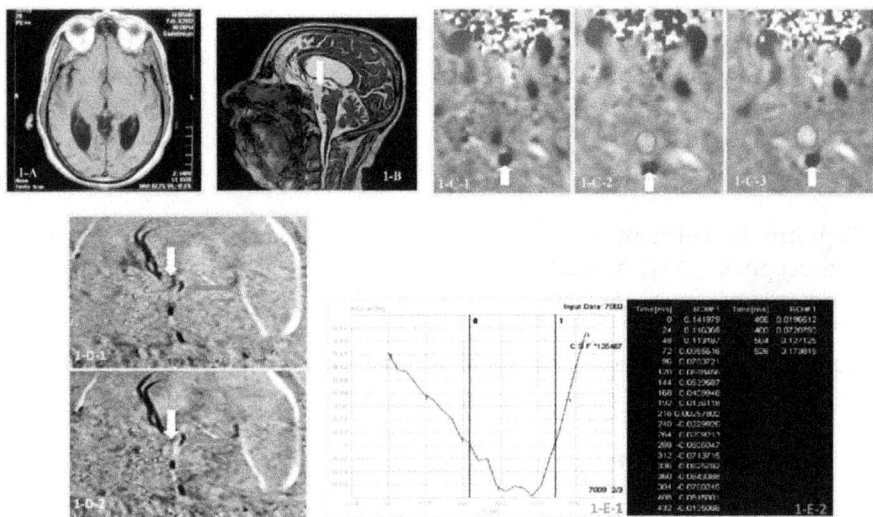

Figure 4.
(A–E): Phase contrast MRI-CSF flowmetry demonstrating a patent endoscopic third ventriculostomy (ETV) stoma with adequate cerebrospinal fluid (CSF) flow in a 62-year-old male patient that underwent colloid cyst resection via ETV. (1-A) Pre-operative axial T1-weighted image shows a colloid cyst in the third ventricle causing obstructive hydrocephalus. (1-B) Post-operative sagittal T2-weighted image demonstrates a floor defect in the third ventricle with the ETV stoma indicated by a white arrow. (1-C1–C3) Axial cine phase contrast MRI images showing the ETV stoma (red circle) with signal changes throughout the cardiac cycle: low signal (black) during systole (1-C1), intermediate during mid-diastole (1-C2), and high signal (white) during peak diastole (1-C3), confirming bidirectional CSF flow; the basilar artery is marked by a white arrow. (1-D1–D2) Mid-sagittal cine phase contrast MRI images showing similar signal transitions at the ETV stoma (white arrow), from systole (1-D1) to diastole (1-D2), again indicating bidirectional flow; the basilar artery is marked by a red arrow. (1-E1–E2) Mean CSF flow curve (1-E1) and corresponding flow values (1-E2) throughout the cardiac cycle, showing the characteristic bidirectional pattern with negative systolic and positive diastolic components, consistent with a patent stoma. Source: Hassanien et al. [15]. License CC BY-NC-ND 4.0.

that up to 85% of individuals with aqueductal stenosis suffer from persistent headaches [16], and 30–50% develop visual disturbances due to papilledema [17].

Additionally, cognitive impairment is seen in 40% of patients, with chronic cases leading to executive dysfunction [17] and memory deficits. Gait instability and coordination deficits, more common in older children and adults, affect 35–50% of cases [16]. If left untreated, these symptoms can severely impact daily functioning, emphasizing the necessity of surgical intervention.

Given its effectiveness in restoring CSF flow without requiring an implanted shunt, ETV is often the recommended surgical approach in these cases [16].

3.3.2 Risk of acute decompensation

A critical factor necessitating urgent surgical intervention is the risk of acute decompensation. In some cases, a sudden CSF flow obstruction due to aqueductal stenosis can trigger rapid neurological decline.

- 10–15% of patients face an acute herniation risk, requiring emergency neurosurgical decompression via ETV or shunting [16].

- 5–10% of patients experience delayed ETV stoma closure, sometimes occurring months or even years after surgery [17].

- 70–80% of untreated patients develop progressive ventriculomegaly, leading to poor neurological outcomes, particularly in neonates and infants (**Figure 5**) [16].

Given these risks, timely surgical intervention is critical in preventing permanent brain damage. For well-selected candidates, ETV remains the first-line approach, providing long-term benefits in reducing shunt dependency [16]. However, the risk of failure and the need for future interventions must always be considered. Successful aqueductal stenosis management relies on early recognition of symptomatic hydrocephalus, identifying treatment-resistant cases, and rapid intervention in acute decompensation scenarios [17].

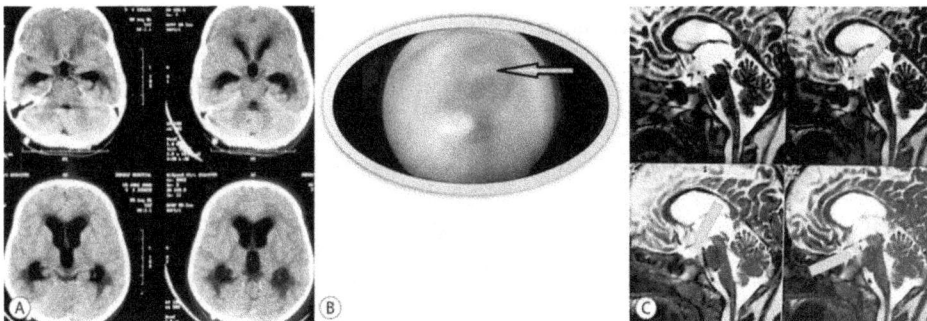

Figure 5.
(A): Primary ETV failure in a child with post tuberculous meningitic hydrocephalus presenting with acute deterioration in emergency. (B): Stenosed stoma with scar in the floor of the third ventricle (arrow) during secondary ETV. (C): MR image showing restoration of CSF flow across the stoma (arrows) post secondary ETV. Patient has not needed any further procedure in 11 years of follow-up with a good intellectual outcome. ETV: endoscopic third ventriculostomy, MR: magnetic resonance, CSF: cerebrospinal fluid, CT: computed tomography. Source: Deopujari et al. [11]. Licensed under CC BY 4.0.

4. Surgical techniques

4.1 Endoscopic third Ventriculostomy (ETV)

Endoscopic third ventriculostomy (ETV) is a widely used surgical technique for obstructive hydrocephalus, particularly in cases of aqueductal stenosis. Unlike ventriculoperitoneal (VP) shunting, which diverts CSF externally, ETV restores natural CSF circulation by creating a bypass in the floor of the third ventricle, allowing direct CSF flow into the interpeduncular and prepontine cisterns [6].

4.1.1 Procedure overview

The procedure is performed under general anesthesia using either a rigid or flexible neuroendoscope. The patient is positioned supine with the head slightly elevated. A burr hole is created at Kocher's point, typically 2–3 cm lateral to the midline and 1 cm anterior to the coronal suture.

Using image guidance, the endoscope is carefully advanced through the foramen of Monro into the third ventricle, ensuring safe perforation while avoiding critical structures such as the mammillary bodies, infundibular recess, and basilar artery (**Figure 6**) [6].

4.1.2 Procedure overview

The ventriculostomy, typically 5–6 mm in diameter, is created at the tuber cinereum using monopolar cautery, a Fogarty balloon catheter, or forceps to prevent premature closure. Free CSF circulation over the stoma confirms procedural success. Once completed, the endoscope is withdrawn, hemostasis is ensured, and the incision is closed.

Postoperatively, careful monitoring is essential to detect complications, including CSF leaks, bleeding, and neurological deficits [18].

4.1.3 Indications and contraindications

4.1.3.1 Indications for ETV

In obstructive (non-communicating) hydrocephalus cases, ETV is the primary indication, especially in:

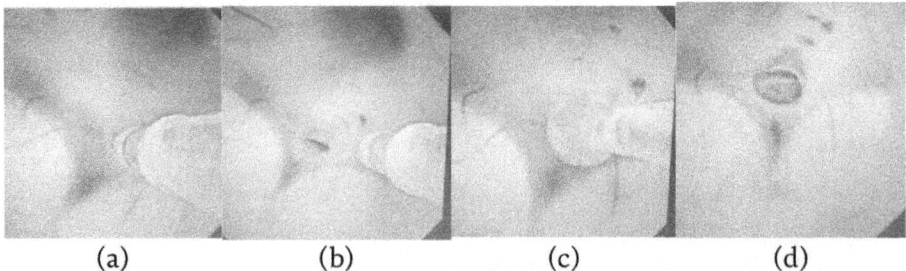

(a)	(b)	(c)	(d)

Figure 6.
From left to write consecutively: (a) Endoscopic visualization of the Liliequist membrane during cauterization (b), Fogarty balloon use during the ventriculostomy perforation step, (c) Final feature showing the opened, and (d) enlarged hole Liliquist membrane in the Floor of the 3rd Ventricle.

- Aqueductal stenosis (whether congenital or acquired)

- Tectal glioma-induced obstructive hydrocephalus

Hydrocephalus due to posterior fossa tumors;
Post-infectious or post-hemorrhagic hydrocephalus associated with an obstruction of the aqueduct.

4.1.3.2 ETV's contraindications

There is no ETV advised in:

- Infants under 6 months due to greater failure rates;

- Communicating hydrocephalus, when CSF absorption is broadly impaired.

- Patients with scarring or adhesions in the prepontine cistern, blocking CSF flow;

- Current infections or coagulopathies, therefore increasing surgical complications [18]

4.1.4 Success rates and failure risk factors

Age, etiology, and past surgical background all affect ETV success rates. Usually, success rates in the first postoperative year range from 50 to 80%.

- Due to an obvious site of obstruction, primary aqueductal stenosis provides the greatest success rate (>75%).

- Immature arachnoid granulates and higher stoma closure risk causes infants under 1 year have fewer success rates (30–50%).

- Adults and older children with aqueductal stenosis have better success rates— between 70 and 85% [6].

ETV potential complications are as follows:

- Stoma closure (5–15%), usually within 6 months after surgery [18].

- 1–3% intraoperative hemorrhage mostly from the basilar artery [6]

- CSF leakage and infections (2–5%), with a 1–2% risk of infection [18]

- Persistent hydrocephalus (10–20%) that requires the transition to VP shunting [18].

In obstructive hydrocephalus, especially in aqueductal stenosis, ETV is nevertheless a safe and successful choice of treatment despite these risks. Advances in neuroendoscopy and intraoperative imaging continue to enhance surgical outcomes, therefore validating ETV as the indicated treatment for non-communicating hydrocephalus [18].

4.2 Ventriculoperitoneal (VP) shunting

VP shunts insertion are among the most common surgeries indicated for hydro-cephalus. In comparison with ETV, that restores normal CSF circulation, VP shunts bypasses normal circulation pathway, directing excessive CSF flow from the ventricles to the peritoneal cavity to be absorbed. Despite its efficacy, VP shunting calls for lifelong monitoring due to its greater potential of long-term complications [19, 20].

4.2.1 Procedure overview

The patient during VP shunting is placed in a supine position, with the head rotated contralaterally for an ideal surgical access.

- For the ventricular catheter placement, a burr hole is drilled at Keen's point.

- After that, the catheter is connected to a programmable or fixed-pressure valve, which serves as a prevention against CSF overdrainage complications.

- A subcutaneous tunnel is created using a trocar, passing from the cranial incision to the paraumbilical region.

- The shunt system is finally tested, the valve connects both catheters, and the peritoneal catheter is inserted into the peritoneal cavity.

4.2.2 Indications and contraindications

4.2.2.1 Indications for VP shunting

VP shunts are indicated when CSF absorption or flow is impaired, such as in the following:

- Communicating hydrocephalus (e.g., post-hemorrhagic, post-infectious, normal-pressure hydrocephalus)

- Obstructive hydrocephalus in which ETV is not possible or failed

- Congenital hydrocephalus which requires long-term CSF shunting

- Hydrocephalus caused by tumors or intracranial hemorrhage [19]

4.2.2.2 Contraindications for VP shunting

VP shunts are not contraindicated in:

- Active central nervous system infections (e.g., bacterial meningitis, ventriculitis)

- Severe peritoneal pathology (e.g., peritonitis, abdominal adhesions impairing CSF absorption)

- Uncontrolled coagulopathy, increasing the risk of hemorrhagic complications [20]

4.2.3 Complications and failure risks

VP shunts' complications are not rare, therefore requiring revisions.

- Shunt malfunction (30–40%), due to disconnection or blockage, which is the most common cause of failure.

- Infections (8–15%), like shunt-related ventriculitis or peritonitis, which may requires shunt removal and external CSF drainage until resolved [20].

- Overdrainage in 10–20% of patients, which leads to slit ventricle syndrome or subdural hematomas.

- Mechanical failure in 5–10% of the cases, due to catheter migration or breakage, may require urgent revision surgery.

- Shunt dependency is also high, with 25–50% requiring revision within the first year and up to 80% of pediatric patients require at least one revision during their lifetime [19].

4.3 Combined and alternative approaches

4.3.1 ETV with choroid plexus cauterization (CPC)

Developed to improve outcomes in high-risk populations, ETV combined with choroid plexus cauterization (CPC) is particularly beneficial for infants under 1 year of age.

- ETV restores CSF circulation, while

- CPC reduces CSF production, thereby increasing long-term success rates [21].

This combined approach enhances the durability of ETV, especially in young patients who traditionally have lower success rates (**Figure 7**).

The approach comprises doing a regular ETV then employing monopolar electro-cautery to coagulate the choroid plexus. Usually targeted at the choroid plexus along the foramina of Monro and the temporal horns to reduce total CSF production, CPC is

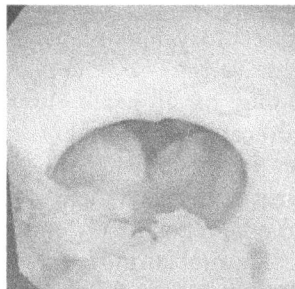

Figure 7.
Endoscopic visualization of the choroid plexus.

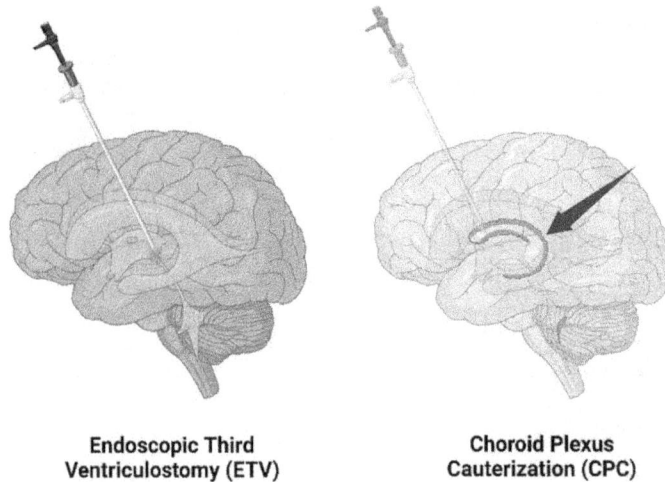

**Endoscopic Third
Ventriculostomy (ETV)**

**Choroid Plexus
Cauterization (CPC)**

Figure 8.
ETV with choroid plexus cauterization CPC.

delivered to the lateral ventricles. Patients with an imbalance between CSF production and absorption—such as those with congenital hydrocephalus (7)—will especially benefit from this method (**Figure 8**).

ETV combined with CPC increases infants' success rates, according to clinical studies, as compared to ETV alone. While adding CPC enhances the chance of sustained success to 50–70% in some cases, the general success rate of ETV alone in children under 1 year of age varies between 30 and 50% [21]. Still, the combined approach is not suitable for every patient. CPC's efficacy relies on the degree of residual CSF absorption capacity; hence, patient selection becomes really essential. Moreover, the procedure includes potential risks such as excessive scarring and poor CSF circulation, which might finally call for shunting [21].

4.3.2 Innovations in minimally invasive techniques

Due to better precision and reduced morbidity, advances in minimally invasive neurosurgery have transformed the treatment of hydrocephalus and CSF-related illnesses. In patient outcomes [22], some newly developed approaches have shown notable benefits. A recent breakthrough is frameless image-guided endoscopy, which integrates neuronavigation devices to improve surgical accuracy. Particularly in situations with distorted ventricular anatomy [22], this method lowers the risk of vascular damage and increases targeting accuracy. Endoscopic-assisted shunt installation is a further advancement that allows real-time catheter placement visualization, therefore lowering the risk of malpositioning and subsequently shunt failure.

Moreover, transforming hydrocephalus treatments are technological developments in neuroendoscopy and robotics. Particularly in patients with complex anatomy [22], robotic-assisted ETV improves precision, hence reducing operational time by 20–30% and limiting complications. When ETV alone is not enough, neuroendoscopic aqueductoplasty has become a substitute for some cases of aqueductal stenosis as it allows direct endoscopic expansion of the aqueduct. Furthermore, flexible neuroendoscopes have reduced tissue disruption [22] and opened surgical access to deep-seated structures.

In pediatric hydrocephalus, especially in infants where shunting is still standard treatment, ETV combined with CPC shows a promising approach. Although it has better success rates than ETV by itself, proper patient selection is still very important. Similarly, developments in minimally invasive techniques—including image-guided endoscopy, robotic-assisted operations, and endoscopic-assisted approaches—continue to hone neurosurgical therapy, thereby lowering complications and increasing long-term outcomes [21, 22].

5. Preoperative and intraoperative considerations

5.1 Preoperative imaging and planning

Evaluation of hydrocephalus is essential on preoperative imaging, which also guides surgical decisions and optimizes results. While neuronavigation technologies improve surgical precision, advanced imaging modalities—especially magnetic resonance imaging (MRI) and cine phase-contrast MRI (PC-MRI)—offer vital insights into cerebrospinal fluid (CSF) dynamics. These tools assist in patient selection, procedure planning, and the detection of anatomical challenges possibly affecting surgical success [6, 14].

5.1.1 MRI and cine phase-contrast studies to evaluate CSF dynamics

Magnetic resonance imaging (MRI) is the gold standard for assessing hydrocephalus and determining the most appropriate surgical approach. High-resolution sequences such as T2-weighted imaging and 3D constructive interference in steady state (CISS) MRI allow for detailed visualization of the ventricular system, aqueductal patency, and periventricular edema [14]. In cases of aqueductal stenosis, MRI enables precise identification of the level of obstruction, which is essential for selecting between endoscopic third ventriculostomy (ETV) and ventriculoperitoneal (VP) shunting [6].

A specialized technique to analyze CSF flow dynamics is cine phase-contrast MRI (PC-MRI), via measuring pulsatile movement in the ventricular system. It is especially used in distinguishing obstructive hydrocephalus from communicating hydrocephalus, assisting in surgical decision-making [14]. Studies have shown that ETV patients with preserved prepontine cistern CSF flow showed significantly higher success rates, indicating the importance of PC-MRI in predicting outcomes [6]. Additionally, PC-MRI has been instrumental in evaluating long-standing overt ventriculomegaly in adults (LOVA), providing valuable insights into altered CSF absorption mechanisms [14, 23].

Further imaging techniques like lumbar infusion tests and nuclear cisternography may be used in patients with complex hydrocephalus or unclear clinical presentation to evaluate CSF dynamics and predict the likelihood of shunt dependency [14].

5.1.2 Role of Neuronavigation

Particularly for endoscopic third ventriculostomy (ETV) and other minimally invasive hydrocephalus therapies, neuronavigation has become an essential tool for modern neurosurgeries. By improving the accuracy of ventricular access, frameless stereotactic neuronavigation reduces the likelihood of complications such as fornix damage, hypothalamus damage, or vascular perforation [6]. When ventricular distortion results from congenital abnormalities, tumors, or prior surgeries, where conventional ana-tomical landmarks may be unreliable [6], this method is extremely beneficial.

The integration of neuronavigation with real-time intraoperative MRI or ultra-sound allows for dynamic tracking of endoscopic instruments, improving precision in ventricular punctures and reducing the risk of catheter malposition [14]. Recent studies show that compared to freehand approaches [6], neuronavigation-guided ETV lowers operational time and increases overall success rates (**Figure 9**).

Beyond ETV, neuronavigation is also crucial for procedures such as aqueducto-plasty, endoscopic cyst fenestration, and biopsy of intraventricular lesions, where spatial orientation within deep brain structures is critical [6]. The combination of preoperative MRI, intraoperative neuronavigation, and advanced imaging modali-ties like PC-MRI is expected to further enhance surgical outcomes in hydrocephalus management, as imaging technologies continue to evolve, [6, 14].

5.2 Anesthetic management

5.2.1 Anesthetic considerations in Pediatric patients

Neonates and infants have a higher baseline cerebral blood flow and reduced cere-brovascular autoregulation, making them more prone to intraoperative intracranial pressure (ICP) fluctuations. Studies have demonstrated that during endoscopic third ventriculostomy (ETV), transient bradycardia and even asystole can occur due to direct mechanical stimulation of the floor of the third ventricle, leading to activation of the vagus nerve [25]. Anesthetic techniques might call for preoperative glycopyrro-late administration and careful intraoperative heart rate and blood pressure monitor-ing to help compensate for that.

Airway management is an additional challenge in pediatric anesthesia, as infants' reduced lung capacities and greater metabolic oxygen needs increase their risk of hypoxia and hypercapnia. Preventing increases in ICP [25] caused by hypercapnia requires controlled breathing with end-tidal CO_2 monitoring. Moreover, pediatric

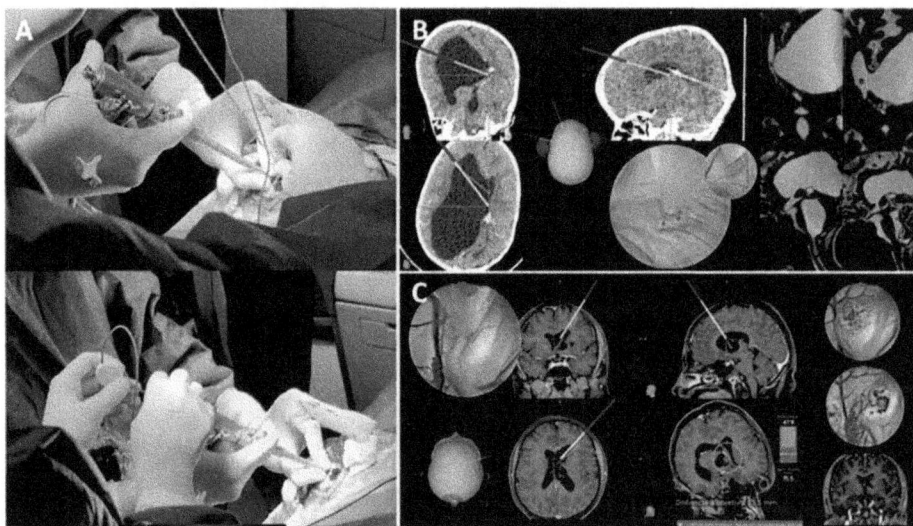

Figure 9.
Navigation of the intraventricular part. Source: Gomar-Alba et al. [24].

patients need cautious dosing of anesthetic drugs due to their immature renal and hepatic metabolism to prevent delayed recovery [14] and prolonged sedation.

Neonates are more prone to hypovolemia and imbalances in electrolytes; hence, intraoperative fluid management is also really important. While too much fluid should be avoided to prevent postoperative cerebral edema [25], isotonic crystalloid solutions are favored to maintain stable hemodynamics.

5.2.2 Anesthetic issues for adult patients

In adult patients, the anesthetic procedure focuses on the risk of thromboembolism, pre-existing comorbidities, and overall cardiovascular stability. Multiple patients undergoing neuroendoscopic surgery have diabetes, hypertension, or persistent hydrocephalus, requiring careful perioperative blood pressure and glucose control [14]. Gradual CSF release and continuous ICP monitoring are particularly crucial, as sudden CSF draining during ETV or ventriculostomy might cause intraoperative hemodynamic instability.

Unlike pediatric cases, adult patients may have higher intracranial compliance, which means their brain can tolerate small volume changes without drastic ICP spikes. However, they remain at risk for venous air embolism (VAE), especially if operated in a semi-sitting position, which is sometimes used for posterior fossa and pineal region endoscopic procedures (**Table 3**) [14].

5.3 Intraoperative challenges and troubleshooting

Endoscopic third ventriculostomy (ETV) is a technically demanding procedure that requires careful intraoperative planning to navigate anatomical variations and manage potential complications. Despite advances in neuroendoscopy, certain challenges—such as distorted ventricular anatomy, vascular proximity, and risk of neural injury—must be anticipated to optimize patient outcomes [6, 26].

5.3.1 Dealing with anatomical variations

Anatomical variations in the third ventricle and surrounding structures significantly impact the feasibility and safety of ETV. One of the primary concerns is

Factor	Pediatric patients	Adult patients
Hemodynamic stability	Prone to bradycardia and asystole due to vagal reflexes during ETV	More stable but at risk of hypertension and hypotension during CSF drainage
Cerebrovascular regulation	Immature, prone to ICP fluctuations	More stable but at risk of vascular complications
Airway management	High risk of hypoxia and hypercapnia	Lower risk but requires monitoring for obstructive sleep apnea (OSA) and aspiration
Fluid management	Requires strict control to avoid dehydration or overload	More tolerable to fluid shifts but at risk of thromboembolic events
Anesthetic agents	Requires lower doses due to immature metabolism	Standard dosing with adjustments for comorbidities

Table 3.
Comparative overview of anesthetic considerations.

Complication	Incidence (%)	Description	Management strategies	Reference
Hemorrhage	1–5%	Intraoperative bleeding, particularly from the basilar artery perforators, can be life-threatening, with severe cases requiring external ventricular drain (EVD) conversion.	Saline irrigation, hemostatic agents, low-pressure tamponade, EVD conversion if needed	[26]
Neural injury	2–5% (up to 10% with memory issues)	Damage to the hypothalamus and fornices can lead to memory impairment, transient disorientation, and endocrine dysfunction such as diabetes insipidus.	Minimize traction, use blunt dissection, avoid excessive perforation force	[6]
CSF leak and pneumocephalus	3–8% (pneumocephalus 4–6%)	Inadequate dural closure can lead to persistent CSF leakage and pneumocephalus, especially in cases of multiple fenestrations.	Dural seal reinforcement, reduced irrigation, fibrin-based sealants	[26]
False passage creation	2–4% (higher in distorted anatomy)	Misplacement of the endoscope due to distorted anatomy or previous surgical scarring can result in injury to the brainstem, optic tracts, or internal capsule.	Neuronavigation, intraoperative ultrasound, careful dissection	[6]

Table 4.
Intraoperative complications and management.

variability in the prepontine cistern, which influences the success of CSF diversion. Studies have shown that a reduced prepontine cistern (<2 mm) correlates with a higher ETV failure rate, making preoperative imaging crucial [6]. Ventricular size and configuration also play a role in procedural success. In cases of long-standing hydrocephalus, the third ventricular floor may become thinned and more transparent, increasing the risk of inadvertent injury during fenestration. In contrast, thicker and more fibrotic floors, often seen in post-infectious hydrocephalus, require greater force for perforation, which raises the risk of hypothalamic injury [6]. Another major variation encountered is basilar artery displacement or aberrant vasculature in the interpeduncular cistern. The proximity of these structures makes endoscopic perforation risky, necessitating gentle blunt dissection techniques and real-time intraoperative adjustments (**Table 4**) [6].

6. Postoperative care and follow-up

In order to optimize outcomes in patients undergoing hydrocephalus surgery, effective postoperative care and long-term follow-up are required. The immediate postoperative period focuses on monitoring for complications, while long-term follow-up evaluates symptom resolution, imaging findings, and potential surgical failures. This section discusses essential postoperative management strategies, including complication prevention, imaging protocols, and approaches for addressing treatment failures [14, 22, 26].

6.1 Immediate postoperative care

Maximizing outcomes following hydrocephalus surgery depends on good postoperative care as well as long-term follow-up. Monitoring complications—including CSF leaks (3–10%), hemorrhage (2–5%), and infections (5–15%)—depends on the 24 to 72-hour immediate postoperative period. Managed with pressure dressings, lumbar drainage, or surgical repair if persistent, CSF leaks may present as rhinorrhea. Hemorrhage calls for rapid CT imaging and, in extreme situations, surgical evacuation; it can lead to sudden neurological impairment. Particularly with VP shunts, infections may require broad-spectrum antibiotics, while shunt infections call for either externalization or removal [22, 26].

Long-term follow-up assesses symptom resolution (headaches, gait, cognition, vision), quality of life, and imaging outcomes. While VP shunt-dependent patients have an increased likelihood of late failure, 70–85% of ETV patients exhibit sustained improvements after 5 years. Given possible learning problems, pediatric patients need neurodevelopmental monitoring. Routine MRI or CT is performed at 3 months, 1 year, and annually to track ventricular expansion, obstructions, and progressive ventriculomegaly. Confirming CSF flow through the stoma in ETV patients is done using cine phase-contrast MRI [14]. With half of pediatric and 30% of adult cases show shunt failure after 2 years, VP shunt patients need lifetime monitoring.

Should surgical failure arise, additional procedures might be required. Early (15–25%) ETV failures arise from inflammatory membrane formation or inadequate perforation, while late failures (5–10%) may require repeat ETV, endoscopic aqueductoplasty, or conversion to VP shunting. Mechanical obstruction (40–50%), infection (15–25%), and overdrainage complications (10–15%) are the most common causes of VP shunt malfunction. Among juvenile shunt patients, up to 80% require at least one revision over their lifetime. Endoscopic-assisted shunt implantation reduces revision rates by 30–40% compared to freehand techniques [26].

7. Outcomes and prognosis

7.1 Comparative outcomes of ETV vs. VP shunting

The two primary surgical approaches for non-communicative hydrocephalus are endoscopic third ventriculostomy (ETV) and ventriculoperitoneal (VP) shunting. Although VP shunting remains the most frequently performed procedure, ETV provides a physiological alternative with better long-term durability in some cases. Short-term outcomes often favor VP shunts due to their immediate effectiveness, although ETV demonstrates superior long-term success, especially in patients with aqueductal stenosis [16]. Studies have shown that combining ETV with choroid plexus cauterization (CPC) significantly improves success rates compared to ETV alone (**Table 5**) [27].

7.2 Prognostic factors

Success of ETV depends on patient age, hydrocephalus etiology, and previous shunt implantation. Studies frequently report that infants under 6 months have far greater failure rates [18], whereas ETV success rates are best in patients with aqueductal stenosis or tectal gliomas and in children older than 2 years. Designed to predict

Parameter	ETV	VP shunting	Reference
Success rate (Overall)	48.6–81.9% (with CPC)	70–80% in short term, declines over time	[18, 27]
Longevity of treatment	Lower early success rate but better long-term durability	High early success but 50% failure at 5 years	[18]
Infection risk	1–5%	10–15% (higher due to implanted hardware)	[18]
Reoperation rate	15–25% (early failure)/5–10% (late failure)	50–80% require at least one revision	[27]
Hospitalization rate	Lower after initial success	Higher due to frequent shunt malfunctions	[18]
Impact on QoL	Improved cognitive and motor development in children	Shunt dependency may cause recurrent hospital visits	[27]

Table 5.
Comparative Overview of ETV vs. VP Shunting.

results based on these factors, the Endoscopic Third Ventriculostomy Success Score (ETVSS) offers a consistent tool that assists in surgical decision-making.

Another essential prognostic factor is surgical time. ETV has a better long-term sustainibility even if its early failure rate is higher [18]. Meta-analyses show that, compared to VP shunting, ETV failure rates generally drop with time. On the other hand, mechanical complications and infections contribute to a cumulative VP shunt failure rate of 50% at 5 years, even if they are initially reliable [18].

7.3 Quality of life considerations

In pediatric cases, the impact of these surgical procedures on the neurological and the developmental outcomes should be taken into consideration. According to studies, children who successfully undergo ETV typically experience better cognitive and motor development compared to those with VP shunts, usually due to avoiding chronic shunt dependency and related complications [27].

Shunt dependency is mostly due to frequent hospitalizations, infections, and hardware failures, which can negatively affect the quality of life on the long term. After 5 years, 81.9% of patients were shunt-free if ETV was combined with CPC, hence reducing the need for recurrent surgeries [27]. Moreover, ETV patients reported less long-term complications—including over-drainage syndromes and infections—than those treated with shunts [18].

Although both surgeries have distinct indications, ETV seems to provide better long-term outcomes in properly selected patients—especially those with aqueductal stenosis. Maximizing treatment results depends on refining patient selection criteria through ongoing research and long-term follow-up examinations.

8. Cases presentation

See (**Table 6**).

Presentation	Imaging findings	Management	Outcome
An 8-year-old boy presented after a minor head trauma with persistent headache, decreased consciousness, vomiting, and ataxic gait.	Fourth ventricular mass extending upward, obstructing the Sylvius aqueduct (**Figure 10**).	Third ventriculostomy (**Figure 11**), followed by posterior fossa craniectomy for tumor resection	Neurological improvement, prepared for definitive tumor resection
A 23-year-old male with persistent headache, visual disturbance, decreased visual acuity, disequilibrium, and inability to focus on daily activities.	Sagittal 3D-CISS image displaying aqueduct Stenosis (**Figure 12**).	Third Ventriculostomy	Complete symptom resolution, returned to daily activities within 2 weeks post-op
A 5-year-old boy with macrocephaly, mental slowness, speech difficulties, and educational difficulties.	MRI imaging displayed congenital aqueductal stenosis (**Figure 13**).	Family opted for VP shunt over third ventriculostomy due to risk concerns.	VP shunt overdrainage led to bilateral subdural hematomas, requiring evacuation and shunt pressure adjustment
A 5-year-old girl with macrocephaly, deafness, and expressive speech aphasia, but no other major symptoms.	MRI brain demonstrated obstructive hydrocephalus secondary to aqueductal stenosis. (a) Axial T1-weighted image, (b) sagittal T1-weighted image with Gadolinium, (c) coronal T1-weighted image postcontrast, and (d) coronal T1-weighted image postcontrast showing the normal sized 4th ventricle (**Figure 14**)	Cochlear implant	Good outcomes in hearing and speech, no surgical indication for hydrocephalus due to absence of intracranial hypertension

Table 6.
Clinical case summaries illustrating diagnostic and surgical management approaches in aqueductal stenosis.

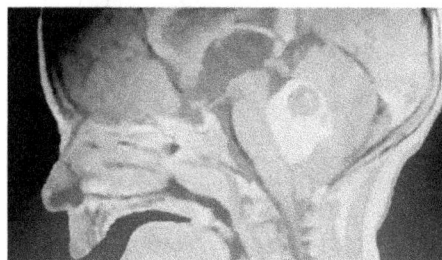

Figure 10.
Sagittal brain CT displaying aqueductal stenosis secondary to a tumor in the fourth ventricle.

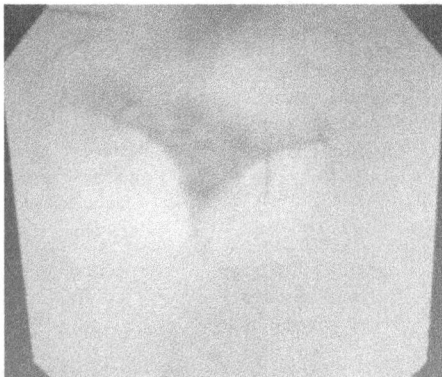

Figure 11.
Endoscopic visualization of Liliequist membrane anterior to the mamillary bodies.

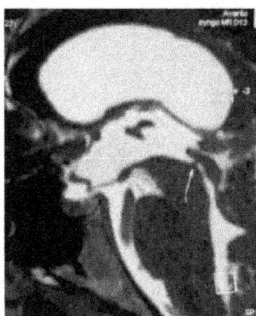

Figure 12.
Sagittal 3D-CISS image displaying aqueduct stenosis.

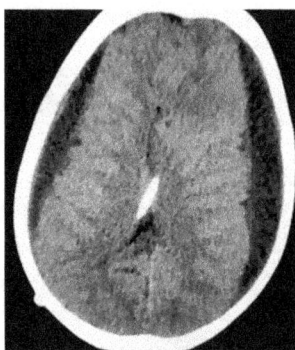

Figure 13.
Shunt malfunction (CT), this axial CT, shows how a shunt overdrainage could lead to ventricular collapse, and sometimes subdural fluid collection which could excacerbate in some cases into subdural hemorrhage and hematoma formation.

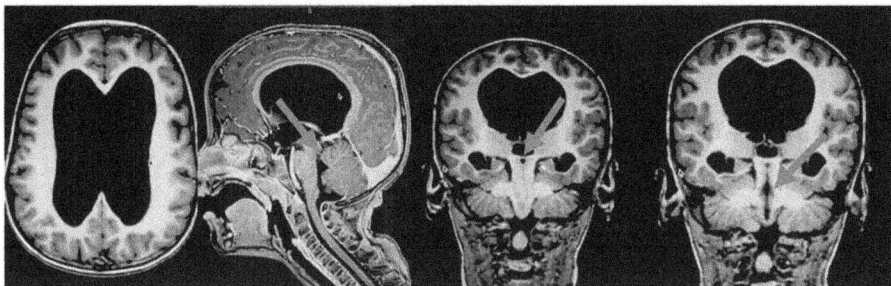

Figure 14.
MRI brain demonstrating obstructive hydrocephalus secondary to aqueductal stenosis. (a) Axial T1-weighted image, (b) sagittal T1-weighted image with gadolinium, (c) coronal T1-weighted image postcontrast, and (d) coronal T1-weighted image postcontrast showing the normal sized 4th ventricle.

9. Challenges and controversies in surgical management

The choice between ETV and VP shunting is challenging in the management of hydrocephalus. While ETV restores normal CSF flow, patient age and hydrocephalus etiology remain important factors influencing its success. In older children and adults, ETV success rates is more than 70% [16] compared to infants under 6 months, where success rates range between 30 and 50%.

While VP shunt insertion procedure provides rapid symptom relief, its failure rate of 50–80% within 10 years often necessitates additional revisions [18]. Though it has limitations—particularly in the case of post-infectious or challenging hydro-cephalus when CSF absorption is impaired—the ETV Success Score (ETVSS) assists with decision-making [27]. Combining ETV with CPC has been found, however, to improve success rates—in some pediatric cases from 80 to 85% [25].

10. Future directions in surgical treatment

The treatment of aqueductal stenosis continues to evolve with innovations in imaging, surgical precision, and biomaterials. Intraoperative MRI and neuronaviga-tion enhance ETV accuracy, enabling safer and more effective perforation of the third ventricular floor [28]. Additionally, robot-assisted neuroendoscopy is being explored to improve precision, reduce operative time, and minimize complications, particu-larly in cases with challenging anatomy [29].

Parallel to these advancements, research in biocompatible shunt materials—including antibiotic-coated and silver-impregnated designs—has demonstrated a 40% reduction in infection rates, addressing one of the primary long-term complications of VP shunting [22]. Additionally, smart shunt systems equipped with pressure sensors and wireless monitoring are under development, offering real-time adjustments to optimize CSF drainage and prevent complications such as over-drainage [30].

Beyond surgical and material innovations, regenerative approaches are being investigated as potential alternatives to shunting. Stem cell-based therapies and molecular treatments targeting CSF production are in experimental stages, showing promise in restoring ependymal integrity and modulating hydrocephalus progression at the choroid plexus level [31]. While still in early development, these approaches represent a potential paradigm shift in hydrocephalus treatment [32]. Future research and multidisciplinary collaboration will be essential in refining these techniques and determining their clinical applicability.

11. Conclusion

The surgical treatment of aqueductal stenosis has evolved so fast and by that offered numerous choices targeted to every case individually. Although endoscopic third ventriculostomy (ETV) is currently the standard treatment in cases of obstructive hydrocephalus, providing a more physiological approach that avoids foreign body implantation, ventriculoperitoneal (VP) shunting remains the standard treatment for patients with impaired CSF absorption. Choroid plexus cauterization (CPC) has added to the indications for ETV, especially in newborns, which enhances long-term success rates in this challenging patient population.

Nevertheless, significant challenges still exist including shunt dependency, ETV failure risks, infection-related issues, and the necessity of frequent surgeries. Improved surgical precision and enhanced outcomes are eased by technological advances such smart shunt systems, intraoperative MRI-guided navigation, and robot-assisted neuroendoscopy. Furthermore, advances in biomaterials including antimicrobial and programmable shunts resolved long-standing problems with infection and over-drainage.

Further research should concentrate on enhancing surgical outcomes by optimizing patient selection criteria, thus reducing surgical complications, and so exploring other approaches other than traditional CSF shunt. By maybe restoring normal CSF dynamics without the need for long-term implants, regenerative therapies—including stem cell-based and molecular approaches—have great potential to profoundly change hydrocephalus therapy.

Continuous innovation, interdisciplinary approaches, and the combined efforts of neurosurgery, bioengineering, and regenerative medicine will guide hydrocephalus therapy moving ahead.

Author details

Mohamed Yazbeck[1*] and Abed Alrazzak Kerhani[2]

1 Department of Neurosurgery, Lebanese Geitawi University Hospital, Beirut, Lebanon

2 Department of Neurosurgery, Klinikum Rechts der Isar, Technische Universität München, Munich, Germany

*Address all correspondence to: mhdyazbeck@gmail.com

IntechOpen

References

[1] Cinalli G, Spennato P, Nastro A, Aliberti F, Trischitta V, Ruggiero C, et al. Hydrocephalus in aqueductal stenosis. Child's Nervous System. 2011;**27**(10):1621-1642. DOI: 10.1007/s00381-011-1546-2. Epub 2011 September 17

[2] Jain K et al. Aqueductal stenosis in pediatric patients: An outcome analysis. Journal of Pediatric Neurology. 2011;**9**(2):187-193. DOI: 10.3233/JPN-2011-0456

[3] Tonetti DA et al. Clinical outcomes of isolated congenital aqueductal stenosis. World Neurosurgery. 2018;**114**:e976-e981. DOI: 10.1016/j.wneu.2018.03.123

[4] Pindrik J et al. Diagnosis and surgical management of neonatal hydrocephalus. Seminars in Pediatric Neurology. 2022;**42**:100969. DOI: 10.1016/j.spen.2022.100969

[5] Gupta D. Neuroanatomy. In: Prabhakar H, editor. Essentials of Neuroanesthesia. Academic Press; 2017

[6] Di Vincenzo J et al. Endoscopic third ventriculostomy: Preoperative considerations and intraoperative strategy based on 300 procedures. Journal of Neurological Surgery Part A. 2014;**75**(1):20-30. DOI: 10.1055/s-0032-1328953

[7] Jung T-Y et al. Prevention of complications in endoscopic third ventriculostomy. Journal of Korean Neurosurgical Society. 2017;**60**(3):282-288. DOI: 10.3340/jkns.2017.0101.014

[8] Byron KYB, Lizano P, Woo TW. Deconstructing the Functional Neuroanatomy of the Choroid Plexus, Research Gate [Accessed: February 4, 2025]

[9] Vitorino Araujo JL et al. Comparative anatomical analysis of the transcallosal-transchoroidal and transcallosal-transforniceal-transchoroidal approaches to the third ventricle. Journal of Neurosurgery. 2017;**127**(1):209-218. DOI: 10.3171/2016.8.JNS16403

[10] Konar SK et al. Neuroendoscopic management of coexisting congenital agenesis of bilateral foramen of Monro with aqueductal stenosis and Chiari malformation: Case report and review of the literature. World Neurosurgery. 2018;**118**:55-58. DOI: 10.1016/j.wneu.2018.07.016

[11] Deopujari CE, Karmarkar VS, Shaikh ST. Endoscopic third Ventriculostomy: Success and failure. Journal of Korean Neurosurgical Association. 2017;**60**(3):306-314. DOI: 10.3340/jkns.2017.0202.013 [Accessed: February 4, 2025]

[12] Rodríguez EM et al. A cell junction pathology of neural stem cells leads to abnormal neurogenesis and hydrocephalus. Biological Research. 2012;**45**(3):231-241

[13] Garg AK et al. Changes in cerebral perfusion hormone profile and cerebrospinal fluid flow across the third ventriculostomy after endoscopic third ventriculostomy in patients with aqueductal stenosis: A prospective study. Journal of Neurosurgery. Pediatrics. 2009;**3**(1):29-36. DOI: 10.3171/2008.10.PEDS08148

[14] Tuniz F et al. Long-standing overt ventriculomegaly in adults (LOVA): Diagnostic aspects, CSF dynamics with

lumbar infusion test and treatment options in a consecutive series with long-term follow-up. World Neurosurgery. 2021;**156**:e30-e40. DOI: 10.1016/j.wneu.2021.08.068

[15] Hassanien O, Abo-Dewan KA, Mahrous OM, Elkheshin S. Evaluation of the patency of endoscopic third ventriculostomy using phase contrast MRI-CSF flowmetry as diagnostic approach. The Egyptian Journal of Radiology and Nuclear Medicine. 2018;**49**(3):701-710. DOI: 10.1016/j.ejrnm.2018.04.004

[16] Rasul FT et al. Is endoscopic third ventriculostomy superior to shunts in patients with non-communicating hydrocephalus? A systematic review and meta-analysis of the evidence. Acta Neurochirurgica. 2013;**155**(5):883-889. DOI: 10.1007/s00701-013-1657-5

[17] Kulkarni AV et al. Outcome of treatment after failed endoscopic third ventriculostomy (ETV) in infants with aqueductal stenosis: Results from the international infant hydrocephalus study (IIHS). Child's Nervous System. 2017;**33**(5):747-752. DOI: 10.1007/s00381-017-3382-5

[18] Labidi M et al. Predicting success of endoscopic third ventriculostomy: Validation of the ETV success score in a mixed population of adult and pediatric patients. Journal of Neurosurgery. 2015;**123**(6):1447-1455. DOI: 10.3171/2014.12.JNS141240

[19] Konar S et al. Endoscopic third ventriculostomy (ETV) or ventriculoperitoneal shunt (VPS) for paediatric hydrocephalus due to primary aqueductal stenosis. Child's Nervous System. 2024;**40**(3):685-693. DOI: 10.1007/s00381-023-06210-w

[20] Kumar P et al. A retrospective study on ventriculoperitoneal shunt complications in a tertiary care Centre CC BY-NC-ND 4.0. Indian Journal of Neurosurgery. 2020;**9**(03):170-174. DOI: 10.1055/s-0040-1713562

[21] Zaben M et al. The efficacy of endoscopic third ventriculostomy in children 1 year of age or younger: A systematic review and meta-analysis. European Journal of Paediatric Neurology. 2020;**26**:7-14. DOI: 10.1016/j.ejpn.2020.02.011

[22] Guillaume DJ. Minimally invasive neurosurgery for cerebrospinal fluid disorders. Neurosurgery Clinics of North America. 2010;**21**(4):653-672. DOI: 10.1016/j.nec.2010.07.005

[23] Kunz M et al. Three-dimensional constructive interference in steady-state magnetic resonance imaging in obstructive hydrocephalus: Relevance for endoscopic third ventriculostomy and clinical results. Journal of Neurosurgery. 2008;**109**(5):931-938. DOI: 10.3171/JNS/2008/109/11/0931

[24] Gomar-Alba M et al. Electromagnetic neuronavigation in neuroendoscopy. Navigation proposal for the LOTTA ventriculoscope. Technical note. Neurocirugía (English Edition). 2025;**36**(1):17-27. DOI: 10.1016/j.neucie.2024.10.003

[25] Furlanetti LL et al. Neuroendoscopic surgery in children: An analysis of 200 consecutive procedures. Arquivos de Neuro-Psiquiatria. 2013;**71**(3):165-170. DOI: 10.1590/s0004-282x2013000300007

[26] Bouras T, Sgouros S. Complications of endoscopic third ventriculostomy: A systematic review. Acta Neurochirurgica. Supplement. 2012;**113**:149-153. DOI: 10.1007/978-3-7091-0923-6_30

[27] Warf BC et al. Long-term outcome for endoscopic third ventriculostomy

alone or in combination with choroid plexus cauterization for congenital aqueductal stenosis in African infants. Journal of Neurosurgery. Pediatrics. 2012;**10**(2):108-111. DOI: 10.3171/2012.4.PEDS1253

[28] Hoshide R et al. Robot-assisted endoscopic third ventriculostomy: Institutional experience in 9 patients. Journal of Neurosurgery. Pediatrics. 2017;**20**(2):125-133. DOI: 10.3171/2017.3.PEDS16636

[29] Bowes AL et al. Neuroendoscopic surgery in children: Does age at intervention influence safety and efficacy? Journal of Neurosurgery. Pediatrics. 2017;**20**(4):324-328. DOI: 10.3171/2017.4.PEDS16488

[30] Tomei KL. The evolution of cerebrospinal fluid shunts: Advances in technology and technique. Pediatric Neurosurgery. 2017;**52**(6):369-380. DOI: 10.1159/000477174

[31] Guerra M. Neural stem cells: Are they the hope of a better life for patients with fetal-onset hydrocephalus? Fluids and Barriers of the CNS. 2014;**11**:7. DOI: 10.1186/2045-8118-11-7

[32] Anwar F et al. Hydrocephalus: An update on latest progress in pathophysiological and therapeutic research. Biomedicine & Pharmacotherapy. 2024;**181**:117702. DOI: 10.1016/j.biopha.2024.117702

Chapter 3

Idiopathic Intracranial Hypertension

*Ravindri Jayasinghe, Nadun Danushka
and Deepal Attanayake*

Abstract

Idiopathic Intracranial Hypertension (IIH) remains a challenging condition characterized by elevated intracranial pressure in the absence of identifiable causes like tumors or venous thrombosis. This chapter provides a comprehensive review of IIH, addressing its increasing prevalence linked to rising obesity rates and the consequent clinical significance. We delve into the complex interplay of factors contributing to IIH's pathogenesis, including cerebrospinal fluid dynamics, venous pressure abnormalities, and metabolic/hormonal influences. The clinical presentation of IIH is discussed, emphasizing the variable nature of headaches, the distressing visual symptoms, and the importance of recognizing papilledema, a hallmark sign. Diagnostic approaches are outlined, highlighting the role of magnetic resonance imaging (MRI) and magnetic resonance venography (MRV) in excluding secondary causes and identifying subtle imaging markers. The chapter explores the association of IIH with systemic diseases, medications, and lifestyle factors, underscoring the need for a holistic approach to patient evaluation. The chapter also addresses various management strategies, including lifestyle modifications, pharmacological interventions, and surgical options tailored to individual patient needs.

Keywords: idiopathic intracranial hypertension, IIH, pseudotumor cerebri, benign intracranial hypertension, increased intracranial hypertension (ICP)

1. Introduction

Idiopathic intracranial hypertension (IIH) is a condition characterized by elevated intracranial pressure without a known cause, distinguished by the absence of an underlying intracranial disorder, meningeal process, or cerebral venous thrombosis [1]. Despite its idiopathic nature, certain conditions such as cerebral transverse venous sinus stenoses and medication-induced cases are still classified under IIH [1]. The term "IIH" is preferred over "pseudotumor cerebri" and "benign intracranial hypertension," as the latter terms can be misleading due to their association with other causes of increased intracranial pressure (ICP) and the potential for irreversible vision loss in IIH patients [2]. Advances in non-invasive imaging have refined our radiological understanding of increased ICP in IIH [3].

IntechOpen

Although idiopathic intracranial hypertension (IIH) is a relatively rare condition, it has become a significant focus of clinical research due to its increasing prevalence, which is closely linked to rising obesity. The incidence of IIH has been observed to rise in various populations worldwide, with notable increases in regions where obesity rates are also escalating. This trend underscores the importance of understanding and addressing the interplay between obesity and IIH to better manage this condition [4].

The pathophysiology of idiopathic intracranial hypertension (IIH) likely involves a complex interplay of multiple mechanisms. These include dysregulation of cerebrospinal fluid (CSF) dynamics, which may involve hypersecretion or reduced absorption, changes in venous sinus pressure that could exacerbate elevated intracranial pressure, and potential metabolic and hormonal factors that are increasingly recognized as contributing elements [5]. The clinical presentation of IIH is characterized by several key symptoms: headache, often severe and chronic; vision loss, which can progress to blindness if untreated; pulsatile tinnitus; and papilledema, the hallmark physical finding. Additionally, some patients may experience cognitive dysfunction1. Understanding these mechanisms is crucial for developing effective treatments to manage symptoms and prevent long-term complications like vision loss. This chapter provides a comprehensive overview of the current evidence of IIH, focusing on the current developments in diagnosis, management and follow-up.

2. Epidemiology

The annual incidence of idiopathic intracranial hypertension (IIH) is generally reported to be between 1 and 2 per 100,000 people in the general population. However, this rate significantly increases among females aged 15 to 44 years who are obese, with incidence rates ranging from approximately 4 to 21 per 100,000. Ireland has one of the highest recorded annual incidences at about 28 cases per 100,000 people [6].

IIH is classically known to occur in overweight females of childbearing age. However, it is known to occur in males, young children, and older adults. These patients with atypical IIH may need further evaluation to rule out other secondary causes [7]. Studies have reported higher frequencies of IIH in those with a family history of IIH and who are obese [8]. Idiopathic intracranial hypertension (IIH) has been associated with several systemic diseases, medications, vitamin deficiencies and excesses, anemia, and hereditary conditions. However, the true relationship between these factors and IIH remains unclear in many instances. While some studies have explored potential links to conditions like menstrual irregularities, pregnancy, antibiotic use, iron deficiency anemia, thyroid dysfunction, and oral contraceptive use, the findings have been inconclusive due to small sample sizes [9].

Among other associations to IIH, several medications and substances have been linked to idiopathic intracranial hypertension (IIH), often supported by temporal associations, resolution with cessation, and recurrence upon rechallenge [10]. Growth hormones, tetracyclines (like minocycline), and retinoids are well-documented examples. Other medications with more limited evidence include thyroid replacement, corticosteroid withdrawal, lithium, and certain antibiotics. Systemic illnesses associated with IIH include obesity-related conditions like sleep apnea and polycystic ovary syndrome, as well as Addison's disease, hypoparathyroidism, anemia, systemic lupus erythematosus (SLE), Behçet syndrome, coagulation disorders, uremia, and vitamin deficiencies or excesses [11, 12].

3. Pathogenesis

Despite numerous theories, the precise pathogenesis of idiopathic intracranial hypertension (IIH) remains unclear. Any proposed etiology must explain the high incidence in obese females of childbearing age. Suggested mechanisms include cerebral venous outflow abnormalities, such as venous stenoses and hypertension; increased CSF outflow resistance at arachnoid granulations or lymphatic drainage sites; obesity-related increased venous pressure both abdominally and intracranially; alterations in sodium and water retention mechanisms; and abnormalities in vitamin A metabolism. These factors likely interact to disrupt cerebrospinal fluid dynamics, leading to elevated intracranial pressure [13].

3.1 Intracranial venous hypertension

Elevated intracranial venous pressure is considered both a primary mechanism and a "final common pathway" for idiopathic intracranial hypertension (IIH). This theory is supported by the similar clinical presentations of IIH and secondary intracranial hypertension caused by cerebral venous thrombosis or other obstructed venous outflow conditions. Some patients initially diagnosed with IIH have later been found to have these conditions, highlighting the importance of differential diagnosis. Studies using magnetic resonance imaging (MRI) and magnetic resonance venography (MRV) have identified cerebral venous outflow abnormalities, such as stenoses, in patients with IIH. However, there is ongoing debate about whether these findings are primary causes or secondary effects of increased intracranial pressure (ICP). Some evidence suggests that elevated ICP can lead to apparent stenosis, which may resolve after interventions like CSF shunting. Conversely, other studies report persistent stenosis despite normalized CSF pressure, leaving open the question of causality [14].

3.2 Increased central venous pressure

Obesity is linked to increased intraabdominal, pleural, cardiac filling, and central venous pressures, which may contribute to elevated intracranial venous pressure and idiopathic intracranial hypertension (IIH). Some evidence supports this theory; for instance, a small study involving obese females with IIH reported symptom relief when using a device that reduced abdominal pressure. However, this mechanism does not fully explain the sex disparity in IIH incidence or its occurrence in non-obese individuals. Despite these limitations, obesity remains a significant risk factor for IIH. Over 90% of patients with IIH are obese or overweight, and the risk of developing IIH increases with higher body mass index (BMI). Weight loss is an effective treatment strategy for managing IIH symptoms2, although the precise pathophysiological link between obesity and elevated ICP remains unclear. Further research is needed to understand how obesity contributes to the development of IIH [15, 16].

3.3 Venous outflow obstruction

Obstruction of venous outflow, such as venous sinus thrombosis, can impair cerebrospinal fluid (CSF) absorption and lead to increased intracranial pressure. This mechanism is observed in conditions like subarachnoid hemorrhage or infectious meningitis, where blockage of arachnoid granulations reduces CSF clearance.

In idiopathic intracranial hypertension (IIH), similar venous outflow obstruction is supported by infusion studies, suggesting that impaired drainage contributes to elevated ICP. However, IIH can also mimic conditions involving CSF overproduction, such as choroid plexus papilloma, highlighting the complexity of its pathophysiology and the need for precise diagnosis to differentiate between these causes.

3.4 Cerebral oedema

Cerebral edema was initially considered a potential mechanism for idiopathic intracranial hypertension (IIH), with some early pathological evidence supporting this theory. However, subsequent studies using both pathological examination and MRI have failed to confirm the presence of cerebral edema in IIH patients. Another proposed link involves altered sodium and water retention. A study found that a significant proportion of IIH patients exhibited peripheral edema and orthostatic sodium and water retention [17]. These patients showed impaired excretion after fluid loading in an upright posture compared to lean IIH patients or obese controls without IIH. Despite these findings, the exact mechanisms connecting orthostatic changes with IIH remain unclear, and many patients do not display these abnormalities [18].

3.5 Hypervitaminosis A

Vitamin A intoxication has been associated with idiopathic intracranial hypertension (IIH) in some case reports, suggesting a potential role for vitamin A in its pathogenesis. Elevated levels of serum vitamin A, retinol, and retinol-binding protein have been observed in some IIH patients. Additionally, studies have found higher concentrations of vitamin A and related compounds in the cerebrospinal fluid (CSF) of IIH patients compared to controls. However, a large case-control study concluded that vitamin A toxicity is unlikely to be a primary cause of IIH [19, 20]; hence, further studies are necessary to establish this relationship.

3.6 Vasodilation secondary to hypercarbia

Obstructive sleep apnea (OSA) is a common comorbidity in patients with idiopathic intracranial hypertension (IIH), particularly due to the shared risk factor of obesity. OSA can potentially contribute to elevated intracranial pressure (ICP) through hypercarbia-induced vasodilation, which may exacerbate IIH symptoms. Studies have shown that a significant proportion of IIH patients experience sleep disturbances, with many having evidence of OSA or upper airway resistance syndrome. While papilledema is rare in sleep apnea patients overall, occurring in about 1% of cases, its presence alongside OSA could indicate a more complex pathophysiological relationship between these conditions and IIH. The prevalence of OSA among IIH patients varies but is notably high. For instance, one study found that nearly half of the women with IIH had obstructive sleep apnea1. The association between OSA and increased ICP during apneic episodes suggests that managing sleep disorders might be beneficial for some IIH patients by reducing intermittent elevations in ICP [21, 22].

3.7 Other factors

Several factors, including leptin and sex hormones, have been explored in the pathophysiology of idiopathic intracranial hypertension (IIH), particularly in relation to obesity. Leptin, a protein secreted by adipose tissue, has been found at higher levels in obese patients with IIH compared to controls. However, the implications of this finding are not well understood. Other studies examining adipokines like leptin and ghrelin have yielded inconsistent results regarding their association with IIH. Sex hormones also play a potential role in IIH. Research suggests that androgen excess may be involved in the condition's pathogenesis, particularly among women with polycystic ovary syndrome (PCOS). In transgender patients undergoing hormone therapy, there is evidence suggesting that exogenous sex hormones could influence IIH development [15]. For instance, some cases report an association between testosterone use and IIH onset. Additionally, studies have identified unique patterns of androgen excess in women with IIH compared to those with PCOS or simple obesity [21, 22].

4. Clinical features

Most patients with IIH are usually overweight females in the childbearing age. The classic symptoms they present would be with headache. However, these symptoms are not specific for IIH individually or as a cluster. Most patients present with headache, transient visual obscurations, pulsatile tinnitus, photopsia, back pain, retrobulbar pain, diplopia, sustained visual loss, and neck pain [23].

Headache is the most common presenting symptom of idiopathic intracranial hypertension (IIH), but its characteristics are variable and not unique to the condition. Many patients experience severe pain, which can be lateralized, throbbing, or pulsatile. Headaches may be intermittent or persistent, occurring daily or less frequently. Associated symptoms include nausea and vomiting, with some patients noting exacerbation with posture changes and relief from nonsteroidal anti-inflammatory drugs (NSAIDs) or rest. Specific features for IIH include retrobulbar pain and mild pain with eye movement. The headache profile often resembles other primary headache disorders like migraine or tension-type headaches, making diagnosis challenging. In some cases, headaches may not occur at all; for instance, in younger children with IIH, headaches are less common than in adults. Men are also less likely to report headaches compared to women. Without headache symptoms, diagnosis often relies on incidental findings of papilledema during routine ocular examinations. The refractory nature of these headaches can lead to medication overuse and rebound headaches, complicating both diagnosis and treatment [24, 25].

Visual symptoms in idiopathic intracranial hypertension (IIH) are significant and can be distressing for patients. Transient visual obscurations occur in about two-thirds of patients, manifesting as brief episodes of blurred or "grayed out" vision, often triggered by changes in posture or Valsalva maneuvers. These episodes are usually not predictive of poor visual outcomes unless they occur frequently. Photopsias, which are brief flashes of light, can also occur and may be provoked by similar factors [26].

Vision loss is a major concern in IIH. Some patients experience rapid progression to severe visual impairment within weeks of symptom onset. This necessitates aggressive treatment to prevent permanent damage. The risk of vision loss is higher in those with more severe papilledema, emphasizing the importance of early diagnosis and intervention. Visual acuity may initially remain normal despite significant visual field defects, making regular perimetry essential for monitoring [27]. Pulsatile tinnitus in the background of headache is a clinical feature of IIH which can be persistent and intermittent and attributed to pulsatile turbulence transmitted through the venous sinuses [28].

The hallmark sign of IIH is papilledema, which involves swelling of the optic discs due to increased intracranial pressure. Papilledema can lead to progressive visual field loss if left untreated. Regular ophthalmologic evaluation is crucial for monitoring the severity and progression of papilledema using scales like the Frisén scale. Additionally, other cranial nerve deficits such as sixth nerve palsy leading to diplopia may occur due to elevated ICP affecting nerves with longer intracranial courses [29].

5. Clinical evaluation and diagnostic approach

IIH is a diagnosis of exclusion. Imaging is usually performed in order to exclude secondary causes for IIH. For diagnosing idiopathic intracranial hypertension (IIH), magnetic resonance imaging (MRI) combined with magnetic resonance venography (MRV) is the preferred diagnostic approach. MRV, especially with contrast, is crucial for detecting cerebral venous thrombosis, which can mimic IIH clinically. While MRI and CT scans typically show normal brain parenchyma and ventricles in IIH patients, certain MRI abnormalities may suggest the condition. These include flattening of the posterior sclera, distension of perioptic subarachnoid space, enhancement of the prelaminar optic nerve with gadolinium, empty sella syndrome, intraocular protrusion of the prelaminar optic nerve, and vertical tortuosity of the orbital optic nerve. Additionally, the narrowing of transverse venous sinuses on MRV is common in IIH patients and supports increased intracranial pressure [30, 31].

Lumbar puncture (LP) is a crucial diagnostic tool for idiopathic intracranial hypertension (IIH), as it measures cerebrospinal fluid (CSF) pressure and analyzes its composition to exclude other causes of elevated intracranial pressure [1]. Accurate measurement of opening pressure requires the patient to be relaxed and in the lateral decubitus position with legs extended; other positions or factors like anxiety can lead to misleading readings. The traditional upper limit of normal for opening pressure is 200 mmH$_2$O, but this may vary, especially in overweight individuals, where pressures up to 250 mmH$_2$O can be considered normal. Interpretation of LP results must consider these nuances. Pressures between 200 and 250 mmH$_2$O are often equivocal, necessitating additional diagnostic support from MRI findings such as transverse sinus stenosis or globe flattening. In young children, higher thresholds are proposed due to variations in baseline pressures among sedated or overweight children. Besides measuring pressure, CSF analysis helps rule out infections or tumors by examining cell count, glucose levels, and protein content. Despite its importance, LP is not without challenges. It is invasive and sometimes painful for patients. Non-invasive methods like transcranial Doppler ultrasonography have been explored as alternatives for estimating intracranial pressure but are not yet widely adopted for definitive diagnosis [2, 32].

Ophthalmologic evaluation is crucial for diagnosing and managing idiopathic intracranial hypertension (IIH). A comprehensive ocular examination should include a formal visual field test, a dilated fundus examination, and optic nerve photographs. Visual field testing is essential to assess the severity of optic nerve involvement and monitor treatment response. Both Goldmann kinetic perimetry and computer-assisted static perimetry are used; the latter is preferred for mild visual loss due to its precision, while Goldmann perimetry is better suited for moderate to advanced cases where variability in results increases [33].

Visual field loss in IIH typically presents as peripheral defects with a predominance of nerve fiber bundle-type abnormalities. Central visual fields may be affected later or earlier if there are concomitant macular pathologies like serous detachment or choroidal folds. The Idiopathic Intracranial Hypertension Treatment Trial (IIHTT) noted common findings such as partial arcuate defects coupled with enlarged blind spots. Generalized constriction of the visual field is also common. In addition to these tests, patients with bilateral optic disc edema should undergo systemic blood pressure measurement to rule out hypertensive retinopathy, which can mimic IIH symptoms. If anemia is suspected, a complete blood count may be necessary to exclude contributory conditions [8, 33].

5.1 Diagnostic criteria

Diagnosis of idiopathic intracranial hypertension (IIH) is primarily based on the modified Dandy criteria. These criteria require the presence of symptoms and signs indicative of increased intracranial pressure, such as headache, transient visual obscurations, pulse synchronous tinnitus, papilledema, and visual loss. Additionally, there should be no other neurologic abnormalities or impaired level of consciousness except for cranial nerve palsies that can occur due to elevated ICP [1].

Elevated intracranial pressure must be confirmed by a lumbar puncture showing normal cerebrospinal fluid (CSF) composition but an elevated opening pressure. Neuroimaging studies like MRI or CT scans are essential to rule out any structural causes for increased ICP such as mass lesions or hydrocephalus. The absence of another identifiable cause for intracranial hypertension is also a critical criterion.

Differential diagnosis is crucial because many conditions can mimic IIH by causing papilledema and increased ICP. Secondary causes include intracranial masses, venous outflow obstruction (e.g., cerebral venous thrombosis), obstructive hydrocephalus, decreased CSF absorption (e.g., post-meningitis), and increased CSF production. Magnetic resonance imaging with magnetic resonance venography is often used to exclude these secondary causes and confirm the diagnosis of IIH when no other etiology is found [34, 35].

6. Management and prognosis

The management of patients with IIH involves two main objectives- management of the symptoms and preservation of vision. Therefore, it is important to identify patients at risk of visual loss and monitor them during treatment. Identifying patients at risk of severe, permanent vision loss in idiopathic intracranial hypertension (IIH) is crucial for timely intervention. Key risk factors include severe papilledema, particularly those categorized as Frisén grades 3 to 5, which indicate a higher risk of poor visual outcomes if not treated aggressively. The absence of papilledema generally suggests a lower risk for vision loss. Significant vision loss at presentation also indicates a higher risk, while transient visual obscurations likely suggest an intermediate level of risk [7, 36].

Other identified risk factors are more variable and include male sex, decreased visual acuity, systemic arterial hypertension, anemia, younger age or onset during puberty, more severe obesity or recent weight gain, and higher opening pressure on lumbar puncture. A subset of patients with IIH experiences a fulminant course characterized by rapid development of vision loss within weeks after symptom onset. These individuals often present with severe papilledema and substantial visual field or acuity loss [37]. In cases where symptoms develop despite treatment or in fulmi-nant disease, aggressive interventions are necessary to prevent permanent vision loss. Such interventions may include surgical options like optic nerve sheath fenestra-tion, ventriculoperitoneal shunting, medical management with acetazolamide, and lifestyle modifications such as weight reduction [26, 38].

Patients with idiopathic intracranial hypertension (IIH) require regular ophthal-mology follow-up visits until their condition stabilizes. The frequency of these visits is tailored to the severity, duration, and response to treatment of clinical manifesta-tions. Initially, patients with moderate symptoms should be seen at least monthly. Those with mild papilledema may require less frequent follow-ups as they are less likely to worsen quickly [39].

Each follow-up visit typically includes a comprehensive assessment: best-corrected visual acuity testing, formal visual field examination, dilated fundus examination with optic disc photographs, and often optical coherence tomography (OCT) of the optic nerve and surrounding structures. These evaluations help monitor for any signs of worsening vision or papilledema progression. If vision deteriorates or symptoms intensify during follow-up, treatment strategies may need to be intensified. Long-term monitoring is essential because IIH can recur even after initial stabilization. Factors such as weight gain can trigger recurrence, emphasizing the importance of ongoing surveillance and adherence to recommended lifestyle modifications like weight management. Regular assessments ensure early detection of potential compli-cations and allow for timely adjustments in management strategies [40].

6.1 Initial management

Initial management of idiopathic intracranial hypertension (IIH) involves addressing modifiable risk factors and comorbid conditions. Discontinuing potential causative agents like tetracycline derivatives is recommended. Polysomnography should be considered to evaluate and treat sleep apnea, as apneic episodes can increase cerebrospinal fluid (CSF) pressure, exacerbating IIH. A low-sodium weight reduction program, ideally with dietary guidance, is crucial for obese patients, as weight loss is associated with reduced intracranial pressure (ICP) and papilledema. For severe obesity, medically supervised programs or bariatric surgery may be neces-sary to achieve significant weight reduction and improve IIH symptoms [39, 41].

For patients with vision loss or symptoms, carbonic anhydrase inhibitors such as acetazolamide are the first-line medical treatment. Acetazolamide reduces the rate of CSF production and has been shown to improve visual fields, papilledema grade, CSF pressure, and quality of life in clinical trials. Dosing should be individualized, starting at 500 mg twice daily and increasing as tolerated up to 2–4 grams per day. Common side effects include paresthesias, anorexia, and electrolyte changes, but these are usually dose-related. Acetazolamide should be used with caution in patients with sulfa allergies and is relatively contraindicated in early pregnancy [42, 43]. For patients who cannot tolerate acetazolamide or require additional treatment, alterna-tive medications include topiramate, which has shown similar efficacy in improving visual fields and relieving symptoms, and other carbonic anhydrase inhibitors like methazolamide. In cases of persistent or worsening visual symptoms despite maximal acetazolamide therapy, the addition of a loop diuretic such as furosemide may be considered [44].

Finally, headache management is an important aspect of IIH treatment. Prophylactic migraine medications can be used to manage headaches that persist despite improvements in papilledema and visual function. Analgesic overuse or rebound headaches should be avoided, and patients should be educated on strategies to prevent this condition [45].

6.2 Urgent presentations

Urgent measures are for patients with fulminant IIH and rapidly progressive visual loss. The objective of treatment is to preserve vision and prevent the progression of visual loss. For patients experiencing acute vision loss due to idiopathic intracranial hypertension (IIH), prompt medical therapy with acetazolamide is essential and can be rapidly increased to a daily dose of up to 4 grams, divided into two administrations. Simultaneously, urgent consultation for surgical intervention is warranted, considering procedures aimed at reducing intracranial pressure and preserving vision. These interventions are typically reserved for severe or refractory cases of IIH [46].

In the period leading up to surgical intervention, short-term measures can be implemented to stabilize the patient's condition. Intravenous glucocorticoids, such as methylprednisolone, may be administered for a brief duration to mitigate acute vision loss, though long-term use is discouraged due to the risk of rebound intracranial pressure elevation. Serial lumbar punctures or continuous lumbar drainage can also serve as temporary strategies to reduce intracranial pressure until more definitive surgical treatment can be performed [47].

6.3 Management of refractory disease

When medical management for idiopathic intracranial hypertension (IIH) fails to prevent worsening visual field defects or visual acuity loss attributed to papilledema, surgical intervention becomes a consideration. These individuals, who have not responded to or cannot tolerate maximal medical therapy, constitute a smaller subset of the overall IIH patient population. While declining vision is a universally accepted indication for surgery, the decision must be balanced against the risks inherent in surgical procedures and uncertainties regarding their effectiveness, particularly when addressing intractable headaches, as the majority of chronic headaches in IIH originate from migraine or other non-intracranial pressure-related causes [48].

The primary surgical options for IIH consist of optic nerve sheath fenestration (ONSF) and cerebrospinal fluid (CSF) shunting procedures. Cerebral venous sinus stenting represents an alternative intervention. Due to the absence of direct comparative studies and variations in indications and outcome measures across case series, the choice of procedure is influenced by local expertise, the availability of surgeons and procedures, and clinician preference. Nevertheless, visual improvement rates appear generally comparable across different surgical modalities. It's worth noting that in some cases, patients might require both shunting and ONSF to achieve optimal outcomes [48–50].

Optic nerve sheath fenestration (ONSF) is deemed an effective procedure for patients experiencing progressive vision loss despite medical therapy. Typically performed using a medial orbital approach, ONSF involves creating a window in the optic nerve sheath to facilitate the drainage of CSF into the orbit. This can stabilize or improve visual loss stemming from papilledema in IIH. Usually conducted as an outpatient procedure under general anesthesia, ONSF primarily aims to preserve vision, and although some patients report headache relief, it's not a universal outcome. It has also demonstrated efficacy in patients whose vision is deteriorating despite a functioning shunt, and it is considered safe and effective for use in children.

Despite its benefits, ONSF carries a complication rate of up to 40 to 45 percent, although most complications are transient and non-disabling [51]. Common complications include temporary diplopia (resulting from injury to extraocular muscles, nerves, or blood supply), efferent pupillary dysfunction (due to ciliary ganglion damage), and vision loss. While vision loss is typically transient, it can be catastrophic and permanent in a small percentage of cases, often due to vascular complications, trauma, infectious optic neuritis, or other operative events. Relapse can also occur following initial benefit, necessitating repeat surgery in some instances [52].

In addition to ONSF, cerebrospinal fluid (CSF) shunting procedures represent a potential alternative or adjunct to surgery for the appropriate patient. Shunting may also be considered when headache or other symptoms such as pulsatile tinnitus are the primary symptom or concern. Shunting involves the placement of a tube to redirect CSF from the lumbar space into the abdomen. Shunting can also be performed with a ventriculoperitoneal shunt where the catheter is directed to the ventricles of the brain. Shunting reduces ICP, and can sometimes result in the resolution of papilledema and improvement in visual symptoms. Shunting is also helpful with refractory headaches [53]. A drawback is that shunts are prone to complications over time including obstruction, infection and over drainage [54–56].

6.4 Other management options

Glucocorticoids, while occasionally employed as a short-term measure before surgical intervention, are generally avoided for the long-term management of idiopathic intracranial hypertension (IIH) due to several concerns. These include the potential for weight gain, which can exacerbate IIH, the risk of severe rebound intracranial hypertension upon steroid withdrawal, and the significant systemic side effects associated with chronic glucocorticoid use [57].

Serial lumbar punctures, despite being advocated by some for IIH treatment, are also generally discouraged due to the rapid reformation of cerebrospinal fluid (CSF), making any benefit short-lived. The procedure is often uncomfortable or painful, carries risks of complications such as low-pressure headaches and CSF leaks, and can be technically challenging in obese patients. However, serial lumbar punctures or lumbar drainage may be considered in pregnant patients seeking to avoid medical therapy [47]. Iron supplementation may be beneficial in IIH patients with iron deficiency anemia [58].

6.5 Prognosis and monitoring

The clinical course of idiopathic intracranial hypertension (IIH) often involves a prolonged duration, typically lasting months to years. Without treatment, symptoms tend to worsen gradually. However, with appropriate treatment, patients generally experience gradual improvement or stabilization of their symptoms. Acetazolamide is commonly used and can be tapered or discontinued once symptoms stabilize. Despite successful management, some patients may continue to experience persistent papilledema and elevated intracranial pressure along with mild residual visual field deficits [59, 60].

Permanent vision loss is a significant concern in IIH but occurs relatively infrequently. Early studies reported higher rates of severe visual impairment compared to more recent outpatient-based research, which suggests a lower incidence ranging from 6 to 14%. Noncompliance with medication is among the risk factors for vision loss. Recurrences are possible in up to 38% of patients after recovery or prolonged stability, often preceded by weight gain. Therefore, long-term monitoring is crucial for managing IIH effectively. Patients should undergo regular follow-ups based on the severity of their papilledema and visual loss history [61]. Patients with Frisén grade 2 papilledema or higher are monitored frequently, typically every few to several months, based on the extent of visual loss and how long their condition has been stable. In contrast, those with chronic Frisén grade 1 edema are examined less often, usually on a yearly or biyearly basis. This less frequent monitoring is justified because the risk of visual loss is relatively low for these patients unless they experience an increase in IIH symptoms [62].

7. Conclusions

Idiopathic intracranial hypertension (IIH) is a diagnosis of exclusion presenting with trivial symptoms that are often neglected, hence, diagnosis of IIH becomes challenging. This sinister pathology in young women of childbearing age can be vision-threatening, and symptoms may cause significant effects on their quality of life. We have explored the epidemiology of IIH, and the potential influence of systemic diseases, medications, and lifestyle factors. Delving into the complex pathogenesis of IIH, we discussed the interplay of factors such as intracranial venous hypertension, central venous pressure, venous outflow obstruction, and the potential roles of identified risk factors. Clinically, IIH presents with a range of symptoms, including headache, visual disturbances, pulsatile tinnitus, and papilledema, necessitating thorough evaluation and diagnosis to rule out secondary causes. Combining the latest research with practical clinical insights, this chapter aims to equip clinicians with the knowledge necessary for accurate diagnosis, effective management, and improved outcomes for patients with IIH.

Acknowledgements

This research did not receive any specific grant from funding agencies in the public, commercial, or not-for-profit sectors.

Conflict of interest

The authors declare no conflict of interest.

Appendices and nomenclature

IIH	Idiopathic Intracranial Hypertension
MRI	Magnetic Resonance Imaging
MRV	Magnetic Resonance Venography
ICP	Intracranial Pressure
CSF	Cerebrospinal Fluid
SLE	Systemic Lupus Erythematosus
BMI	Body Mass Index

OSA	Obstructive Sleep Apnea
PCOS	Polycystic Ovoru Syndrome
NSAIDs	Non-Steroidal Anti-Inflammatory Drugs
LP	Lumbar Puncture
IIHTT	Idiopathic Intracranial Hypertension Treatment Trial
CT	Computed Tomography
OCT	Optical Coherance Tomography
ONSF	Optic Nerve Sheath Fenestration

Declaration

There are no additional declarations for this manuscript.

Author details

Ravindri Jayasinghe, Nadun Danushka* and Deepal Attanayake
Department of Neurosurgery, National Hospital of Sri Lanka, Sri Lanka

*Address all correspondence to: danupiti@gmail.com

IntechOpen

References

[1] Friedman DI, Jacobson DM. Diagnostic criteria for idiopathic intracranial hypertension. Neurology. 2002;**59**(10):1492-1495

[2] Farb R, Vanek I, Scott J, Mikulis D, Willinsky R, Tomlinson G, et al. Idiopathic intracranial hypertension: The prevalence and morphology of sinovenous stenosis. Neurology. 2003;**60**(9):1418-1424

[3] Kapoor KG. More than meets the eye? Redefining idiopathic intracranial hypertension. International Journal of Neuroscience. 2010;**120**(7):471-482

[4] St MI, Iencean AS, Tascu A. Pseudotumour cerebri: Idiopathic intracranial hypertension and vascular intracranial hyertension. Romanian Neurosurgery. 2015;**XXIX**(4):397-409

[5] Wang MT, Bhatti MT, Danesh-Meyer HV. Idiopathic intracranial hypertension: Pathophysiology, diagnosis and management. Journal of Clinical Neuroscience. 2022;**95**:172-179

[6] Durcan FJ, Corbett JJ, Wall M. The incidence of pseudotumor cerebri: Population studies in Iowa and Louisiana. Archives of Neurology. 1988;**45**(8):875-877

[7] Bruce B, Kedar S, Van Stavern G, Corbett J, Newman N, Biousse V. Atypical idiopathic intracranial hypertension: Normal BMI and older patients. Neurology. 2010;**74**(22):1827-1832

[8] Wall M, Kupersmith MJ, Kieburtz KD, Corbett JJ, Feldon SE, Friedman DI, et al. The idiopathic intracranial hypertension treatment trial: Clinical

profile at baseline. JAMA Neurology. 2014;**71**(6):693-701

[9] Giuseffi V, Wall M, Siegel PZ, Rojas PB. Symptoms and disease associations in idiopathic intracranial hypertension (pseudotumor cerebri) a case-control study. Neurology. 1991;**41**(2_part_1):239

[10] Friedman DI. Medication-induced intracranial hypertension in dermatology. American Journal of Clinical Dermatology. 2005;**6**:29-37

[11] Sussman J, Leach M, Greaves M, Malia R, Davies-Jones G. Potentially prothrombotic abnormalities of coagulation in benign intracranial hypertension. Journal of Neurology, Neurosurgery & Psychiatry. 1997;**62**(3):229-233

[12] Glueck CJ, Iyengar S, Goldenberg N, Smith L-S, Wang P. Idiopathic intracranial hypertension: Associations with coagulation disorders and polycystic-ovary syndrome. Journal of Laboratory and Clinical Medicine. 2003;**142**(1):35-45

[13] Biousse V, Bruce BB, Newman NJ. Update on the pathophysiology and management of idiopathic intracranial hypertension. Journal of Neurology, Neurosurgery & Psychiatry. 2012;**83**(5):488-494

[14] Biousse V, Ameri A, Bousser M-G. Isolated intracranial hypertension as the only sign of cerebral venous thrombosis. Neurology. 1999;**53**(7):1537

[15] Sugerman H, DeMaria E, Felton Iii W, Nakatsuka M, Sismanis A. Increased intra-abdominal pressure and cardiac filling pressures in

obesity-associated pseudotumor cerebri. Neurology. 1997;**49**(2):507-511

[16] Friedman DI. Cerebral venous pressure, intra-abdominal pressure, and dural venous sinus stenting in idiopathic intracranial hypertension. Journal of Neuro-Ophthalmology. 2006;**26**(1):61-64

[17] Wall M, Dollar JD, Sadun AA, Kardon R. Idiopathic intracranial hypertension: Lack of histologic evidence for cerebral edema. Archives of Neurology. 1995;**52**(2):141-145

[18] Owler B, Higgins J, Péna A, Carpenter T, Pickard J. Diffusion tensor imaging of benign intracranial hypertension: Absence of cerebral edema. British Journal of Neurosurgery. 2006;**20**(2):79-81

[19] Warner JE, Bernstein PS, Yemelyanov A, Alder SC, Farnsworth ST, Digre KB. Vitamin a in the cerebrospinal fluid of patients with and without idiopathic intracranial hypertension. Annals of Neurology: Official Journal of the American Neurological Association and the Child Neurology Society. 2002;**52**(5):647-650

[20] Tabassi A, Salmasi AH, Jalali M. Serum and CSF vitamin a concentrations in idiopathic intracranial hypertension. Neurology. 2005;**64**(11):1893-1896

[21] Ooi L-Y, Walker B, Bodkin P, Whittle I. Idiopathic intracranial hypertension: Can studies of obesity provide the key to understanding pathogenesis? British Journal of Neurosurgery. 2008;**22**(2):187-194

[22] Subramanian PS, Goldenberg-Cohen N, Shukla S, Cheskin LJ, Miller NR. Plasma ghrelin levels are normal in obese patients with idiopathic intracranial hypertension (pseudotumor

cerebri). American Journal of Ophthalmology. 2004;**138**(1):109-113

[23] Wall M, GEORGE D. Idiopathic intracranial hypertension: A prospective study of 50 patients. Brain. 1991;**114**(1):155-180

[24] Wall M. The headache profile of idiopathic intracranial hypertension. Cephalalgia. 1990;**10**(6):331-335

[25] Quattrone A, Bono F, Fera F, Lavano A. Isolated unilateral abducens palsy in idiopathic hypertension without papilledema. European Journal of Neurology. 2006;**13**:670-671

[26] Thambisetty M, Lavin PJ, Newman NJ, Biousse V. Fulminant idiopathic intracranial hypertension. Neurology. 2007;**68**(3):229-232

[27] Liu GT, Glaser JS, Schatz NJ. High-dose methylprednisolone and acetazolamide for visual loss in pseudotumor cerebri. American Journal of Ophthalmology. 1994;**118**(1):88-96

[28] Sismanis A, Butts FM, Hughes GB. Objective tinnitus in benign intracranial hypertension: An update. Laryngoscope. 1990;**100**(1):33-36

[29] Lim M, Kurian M, Penn A, Calver D, Lin J. Visual failure without headache in idiopathic intracranial hypertension. Archives of Disease in Childhood. 2005;**90**(2):206-210

[30] Lin A, Foroozan R, Danesh-Meyer HV, De Salvo G, Savino PJ, Sergott RC. Occurrence of cerebral venous sinus thrombosis in patients with presumed idiopathic intracranial hypertension. Ophthalmology. 2006;**113**(12):2281-2284

[31] Yuh WT, Zhu M, Taoka T, Quets JP, Maley JE, Muhonen MG, et al. MR

imaging of pituitary morphology in idiopathic intracranial hypertension. Journal of Magnetic Resonance Imaging. 2000;**12**(6):808-813

[32] Torbey M, Geocadin R, Razumovsky A, Rigamonti D, Williams M. Utility of CSF pressure monitoring to identify idiopathic intracranial hypertension without papilledema in patients with chronic daily headache. Cephalalgia. 2004;**24**(6):495-502

[33] Wall M, George D. Visual loss in pseudotumor cerebri: Incidence and defects related to visual field strategy. Archives of Neurology. 1987;**44**(2):170-175

[34] Sylaja P, Moosa NA, Radhakrishnan K, Sarma PS, Kumar SP. Differential diagnosis of patients with intracranial sinus venous thrombosis related isolated intracranial hypertension from those with idiopathic intracranial hypertension. Journal of the Neurological Sciences. 2003;**215**(1-2):9-12

[35] Leker RR, Steiner I. Features of dural sinus thrombosis simulating pseudotumor cerebri. European Journal of Neurology. 1999;**6**(5):601-604

[36] Corbett JJ, Savino PJ, Thompson HS, Kansu T, Schatz NJ, Orr LS, et al. Visual loss in pseudotumor cerebri: Follow-up of 57 patients from five to 41 years and a profile of 14 patients with permanent severe visual loss. Archives of Neurology. 1982;**39**(8):461-474

[37] Wall M, Falardeau J, Fletcher WA, Granadier RJ, Lam BL, Longmuir RA, et al. Risk factors for poor visual outcome in patients with idiopathic intracranial hypertension. Neurology. 2015;**85**(9):799-805

[38] Kidron D, Pomeranz S. Malignant pseudotumor cerebri: Report of two cases. Journal of Neurosurgery. 1989;**71**(3):443-445

[39] Wall M, McDermott MP, Kieburtz KD, Corbett JJ, Feldon SE, Friedman DI, et al. Effect of acetazolamide on visual function in patients with idiopathic intracranial hypertension and mild visual loss: The idiopathic intracranial hypertension treatment trial. JAMA. 2014;**311**(16):1641-1651

[40] Wall M. Sensory visual testing in idiopathic intracranial hypertension: Measures sensitive to change. Neurology. 1990;**40**(12):1859

[41] Sinclair AJ, Burdon MA, Nightingale PG, Ball AK, Good P, Matthews TD, et al. Low energy diet and intracranial pressure in women with idiopathic intracranial hypertension: Prospective cohort study. BMJ. 2010;**341**

[42] Krajnc N, Itariu B, Macher S, Marik W, Harreiter J, Michl M, et al. Treatment with GLP-1 receptor agonists is associated with significant weight loss and favorable headache outcomes in idiopathic intracranial hypertension. The Journal of Headache and Pain. 2023;**24**(1):89

[43] Chandra V, Dutta S, Albanese CT, Shepard E, Farrales-Nguyen S, Morton J. Clinical resolution of severely symptomatic pseudotumor cerebri after gastric bypass in an adolescent. Surgery for Obesity and Related Diseases. 2007;**3**(2):198-200

[44] Lee AG, Pless M, Falardeau J, Capozzoli T, Wall M, Kardon RH. The use of acetazolamide in idiopathic intracranial hypertension during pregnancy. American Journal of Ophthalmology. 2005;**139**(5):855-859

[45] Friedman DI, Rausch EA. Headache diagnoses in patients with treated idiopathic intracranial hypertension. Neurology. 2002;**58**(10):1551-1553

[46] Hunt J, Olivieri P. Recognizing and managing idiopathic intracranial hypertension in the emergency department. Current Emergency and Hospital Medicine Reports. 2023;**11**(3):126-132

[47] Huna-Baron R, Kupersmith MJ. Idiopathic intracranial hypertension in pregnancy. Journal of Neurology. 2002;**249**:1078-1081

[48] Fonseca PL, Rigamonti D, Miller NR, Subramanian PS. Visual outcomes of surgical intervention for pseudotumour cerebri: Optic nerve sheath fenestration versus cerebrospinal fluid diversion. British Journal of Ophthalmology. 2014;**98**(10):1360-1363

[49] Spitze A, Lam P, Al-Zubidi N, Yalamanchili S, Lee AG. Controversies: Optic nerve sheath fenestration versus shunt placement for the treatment of idiopathic intracranial hypertension. Indian Journal of Ophthalmology. 2014;**62**(10):1015-1021

[50] Lai LT, Danesh-Meyer HV, Kaye AH. Visual outcomes and headache following interventions for idiopathic intracranial hypertension. Journal of Clinical Neuroscience. 2014;**21**(10):1670-1678

[51] Plotnik JL, Kosmorsky GS. Operative complications of optic nerve sheath decompression. Ophthalmology. 1993;**100**(5):683-690

[52] Chandrasekaran S, McCluskey P, Minassian D, Assaad N. Visual outcomes for optic nerve sheath fenestration in pseudotumour cerebri and related conditions. Clinical & Experimental Ophthalmology. 2006;**34**(7):661-665

[53] Johnston I, Besser M, Morgan MK. Cerebrospinal fluid diversion in the treatment of benign intracranial hypertension. Journal of Neurosurgery. 1988;**69**(2):195-202

[54] McGirt MJ, Woodworth G, Thomas G, Miller N, Williams M, Rigamonti D. Cerebrospinal fluid shunt placement for pseudotumor cerebri—Associated intractable headache: Predictors of treatment response and an analysis of long-term outcomes. Journal of Neurosurgery. 2004;**101**(4):627-632

[55] Suri A, Pandey P, Mehta V. Subarachnoid hemorrhage and intracereebral hematoma following lumboperitoneal shunt for pseudotumor cerebri: A rare complication. Neurology India. 2002;**50**(4):508-510

[56] Ahmed R, Wilkinson M, Parker G, Thurtell M, Macdonald J, McCluskey P, et al. Transverse sinus stenting for idiopathic intracranial hypertension: A review of 52 patients and of model predictions. American Journal of Neuroradiology. 2011;**32**(8):1408-1414

[57] Friedman DI, Jacobson DM. Idiopathic intracranial hypertension. Journal of Neuro-Ophthalmology. 2004;**24**(2):138-145

[58] Biousse V, Rucker JC, Vignal C, Crassard I, Katz BJ, Newman NJ. Anemia and papilledema. American Journal of Ophthalmology. 2003;**135**(4):437-446

[59] Celebisoy N, Secil Y, Akyürekli Ö. Pseudotumor cerebri: Etiological factors, presenting features and prognosis in the western part of Turkey. Acta Neurologica Scandinavica. 2002;**106**(6):367-370

[60] Bruce BB, Preechawat P, Newman NJ, Lynn MJ, Biousse V. Racial differences in idiopathic

intracranial hypertension. Neurology.
2008;**70**(11):861-867

[61] Wall M, Johnson CA, Cello KE,
Zamba KD, McDermott MP, Keltner JL,
et al. Visual field outcomes for the
idiopathic intracranial hypertension
treatment trial (IIHTT). Investigative
Ophthalmology & Visual Science.
2016;**57**(3):805-812. DOI: 10.1167/
iovs.15-18626

[62] Wall M, Lee AG, Swanson JW,
Wilterdink JL. Idiopathic Intracranial
Hypertension (Pseudotumor Cerebri):
Prognosis and Treatment. Waltham, MA,
USA: UpToDate; 2017

Chapter 4

Complications of Ventriculoperitoneal Shunt Surgery

Aliyu Muhammad Koko and Muhammad Mansur Idris

Abstract

Hydrocephalus is one of the commonest neurosurgical pathologies encountered by neurosurgeons in clinical practice. Ventriculoperitoneal shunt (VPS) remains the most popular surgical treatment option for hydrocephalus. Complications do occur following VPS and are of a wide spectrum and can involve any anatomical area along the path of ventriculoperitoneal shunt. Complications could affect any age group, but children are more prone to these unwanted events. Complications of ventriculoperitoneal shunt surgery were categorised based on the anatomical segment of the body involved into cranial, cervico-thoracic, and abdominal. Generally, shunt obstruction is the commonest complication and could affect any part of the shunt catheter. Detailed information on specific complications was outlined, including treatment strategies. Careful patient and shunt selection and surgical technique will help in preventing shunt complications and improving the health and well-being of hydrocephalic patients.

Keywords: ventriculoperitoneal shunt, shunt obstruction, shunt infection, CSF shunt metastasis, silicon reaction

1. Introduction

Ventriculoperitoneal shunt (VPS) remains a common neurosurgical procedure globally. It is offered to a wide spectrum of patients with hydrocephalus across all age groups, from the neonatal period to the elderly. Complications do arise from VPS, leading to the reversal of signs and symptoms of hydrocephalus or worsening the clinical states of patients before surgery was carried out. Ventriculoperitoneal shunt complications occur more often in patients within the first year of surgery and seen in 17-33% of ventriculoperitoneal shunt surgeries [1, 2]. Shunt obstruction and shunt infections are the most frequent causes of shunt failure, with infections accounting for early shunt failure while obstruction being responsible for late shunt failures [3–5]. Shunt complications continue to result in recurrent hospital admissions, shunt revisions, and replacements amounting to huge amounts of medical costs for the management of hydrocephalus. Various measures to prevent the occurrence of shunt complications have been developed, such as the use of programmable shunts and antibiotic-impregnated shunts, but these unwanted events still persist in hydrocephalic patients treated by shunting.

Shunt complications can be classified based on the anatomical area involved into: cranial, cervico-thoracic, and abdominal.

2. Cranial complications

1. Proximal shunt obstruction

2. Shunt infection

3. Seizure

4. Shunt migration outside the ventricles

5. Intraparenchymal and intraventricular haemorrhages

6. Antegrade and retrograde CSF shunt metastasis

7. Craniosynostosis and skull deformity

3. Cervico-thoracic complications

1. Shunt tract infection

2. Shunt calcification

3. Valve dysfunction leading to over or under shunting

4. Retrograde metastatic deposits.

5. Shuntalgia

4. Abdomianal complications

1. Distal shunt obstruction

2. Shunt infection

3. Shunt viscus perforation and extrusion via mouth, anus, vagina

4. Shunt ascites

5. Pseudocyst

6. Antegrade CSF shunt metastasis

5. Risk factors for shunt complications

1. Neonatal period [1]

2. Male gender

3. Low socioeconomic factors

4. Paediatric age group 4 times compared to adult

5. Congenital hydrocephalus

6. Associated spinal dysraphism

7. Previous abdominal surgery before shunt

6. Methodology

This is a review of relevant literature discussing various complications of ventriculoperitoneal shunt surgery. Inclusion criteria were papers published on specific complications of ventriculoperitoneal shunt from 1954 to 2025. Ventriculoatrial and pleural were excluded.

7. Obstruction

Ventriculoperitoneal shunt obstruction is defined as the blockage of VPS tubing, hindering the normal flow of cerebrospinal fluid from the ventricles of the brain to the peritoneum. It is the commonest cause of shunt failure [3]. Shunt obstruction could occur at any part of the shunt from the proximal catheter, within the valve, and the distal catheter, but proximal obstruction remains the most affected [3]. Possible causes of proximal shunt obstruction include clogging with brain parenchyma as the catheter passes through the brain, pieces of choroid plexus, and debris from haemorrhage or protein-rich fluid within the ventricles. Distal shunt obstruction may result from blockage of distal opening by omentum, trapping of debris within the shunt system, peritoneal cyst, omentum as "policeman of the abdomen" may wall off a nidus of irritation from talc in surgical gloves or infection of the peritoneum and eventually blocked the distal opening of the shunt tubing. In addition, misplacement of catheter tip in preperitoneal fat during surgery contributes to distal catheter occlusion. Patients with shunt obstruction are present with headache, nausea, vomiting, and lethargy, and other features of raised intracranial pressure depending on the duration and severity of shunt obstruction. Regarding the severity of shunt obstruction, in some instances the shunt opening may be partially occluded, thereby presenting with reduced drainage and subtle features of hydrocephalus compared to a more severe form of complete occlusion of shunt. Also, individuals who present weeks after the development of features of shunt obstruction tend to have more severe and chronic features of hydrocephalus. The level of shunt obstruction can be determined by assessing the CSF flow and valve refilling after digital pressure over the valve. Shunt valve becomes incompressible when there is distal catheter obstruction, while in proximal catheter occlusion, the valve collapses following digital pressure, displacing the remaining CSF within it and does not refill. Other relevant evaluations that may unravel the site and extent of shunt obstruction include shunt series, brain CT scans, and radionuclide studies, as well as shunt tapping.

8. Infection

Shunt infection is a common complication of ventriculoperitoneal shunt; it's the second most common complication after obstruction. The incidence of shunt infection was reported to be 5–47% [1, 3, 4]. The risk factors for shunt infection identified include young age (neonatal period), presence of post-operative CSF leak, previous infections, intraventricular haemorrhage. The causative organisms commonly implicated include staph epidermidis, staph aureus, and gram-negative rods [1, 5]. Patients with shunt infection present with excessive crying or headache, nausea, vomiting, and fever. Infection localised to the brain and ventricles are more severe and patients may have altered conscious level and usually acutely sick. The presence of erythema and tenderness along the shunt in the neck, chest, and anterior abdominal wall may serve as a pointer to shunt infection. Distal or peritoneal catheter infection usually have localised or generalised abdominal pain and tenderness. CSF tapped from shunt tubing or valve may be turbid and have debris. CSF culture could reveal offending organisms, where culture is negative in most cases as patients could be on antibiotics. Polymerase chain reaction can detect the DNA or RNA of an organism even in negative culture; as such, it is recommended when culture is not helpful. The presence of >10% neutrophils in CSF has high sensitivity and specificity in detecting shunt infection. Treatments for shunt infection include removal of the infected shunt, externalising it, or complete removal of the shunt and placement of an external ventricular drain plus intravenous antibiotic therapy. In patients with active hydrocephalus, a repeat shunt can be done from 6 weeks to 3 months after treatment of shunt infection. Measures to prevent shunt infection include use of antibiotic-impregnated shunts (reduces risk of infection from 6 to 2.2%), perioperative antibiotics, ensuring optimal sterile technique and skin preparation, and reduction of operating time to a minimum [6]. In some centres where antibiotic-impregnated shunt is unavailable, shunt tubing is inserted into gentamycin solution as soon as it's removed from the pack till complete placement in the ventricle and the peritoneum. Shunt infection causes increasing morbidity and mortality in hydrocephalic patients, prolong duration of hospital stay, reduces IQ and significantly add to the cost of management of hydrocephalus (**Figure 1**).

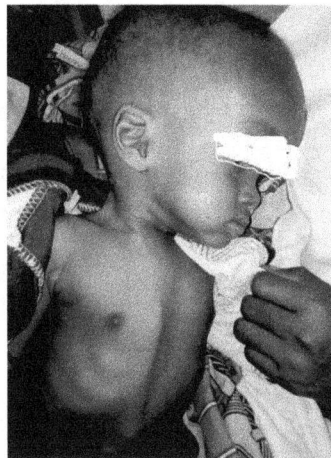

Figure 1.
An infant with shunt tract infection as evidence by erythema along the tract.

9. Abdominal CSF pseudocyst

Abdominal pseudocyst is described as the collection of CSF around the tip of the peritoneal catheter surrounded by a wall of fibrous tissue with no epithelial lining. It is a rare late complication of ventriculoperitoneal shunt occurring in 1–4.5% of cases, usually seen a year or more after VP shunting. First reported by Harsh in 1954 [3, 6]. Pseudocysts occur as a result of infection or allergic reaction to peritoneal catheter with subsequent inflammation and adhesions around the catheter tip in the abdominal cavity. High CSF protein and liver dysfunction have been found to contribute to formation of pseudocyst [3, 7, 8]. Hepatic CSF pseudocyst may occur when a peritoneal catheter migrates to the surface of the liver, causing irritation, inflammation, and consequent pseudocyst formation [3]. Presentation of abdominal pseudocyst depends on location in the abdomen but usually is present with pain, distension, and abdominal mass. In hepatic pseudocyst, elevated liver enzymes may occur. Abdominal ultrasound or CT scan will reveal the site of the pseudocyst, its size, and the nature of the surrounding structures and may give a clue to a likely infection within the cyst. Treatment of pseudocyst depends on whether infection of shunt catheter is established or not as well as experience of the surgeon. Where there is shunt infection, the shunt should be externalised, laparotomy and excision of the pseudocyst offered. In the absence of infection, the peritoneal catheter should be repositioned into other spaces like ventriculo-pleural or ventriculoatrial. Following CSF diversion to non-peritoneal spaces, CT or ultrasound-guided aspiration of pseudocyst may suffice and avoid the need for laparotomy and cyst excision, which is more invasive. It's believed that CSF diversion allows for cyst reabsorption, thus making cyst excision unnecessary. Recurrence of pseudocyst is lower in children and those whose CSF diverted to non-peritoneal spaces.

10. Shunt perforation

Bowel perforation is an uncommon complication of VP shunting, occurring in 0.1–0.7% [1]. Factors associated with bowel perforation include the sharp tip of the peritoneal catheter, presence of infection, higher CSF protein, frictional force of the shunt and silicon allergy, congenital hydrocephalus, and coexisting myelomeningocele [3]. Bowel perforation may occur immediately following shunt catheter insertion or months later. The presentation of shunt bowel perforation includes extrusion via anus or oral cavity, unexplained diarrhoea or abdominal pain, and meningitis caused by gram-negative bacilli. Peritonitis is not common in bowel perforation caused by a shunt catheter, as the site of perforation is small and walled by fibrosed tissues. The presence of meningitis or peritonitis accounts for mortality of 15% seen in the shunt-related bowel perforation [3, 9]. Treatment of bowel perforation include removal of shunt, co-management of abdominal features with paediatric surgeons and subsequent shunt insertion at 6 weeks or 3 months after abdominal symptoms cleared. Ventriculoperitoneal shunt can be done, though there is higher chance of abdominal complications like pseudocyst, distal catheter occlusion from possible infection, inflammation and adhesions that might have occurred.

11. CSF ascites

CSF ascites is defined as the pathologic accumulation of CSF within the peritoneal cavity. It's also called CSF hydroperitoneum. CSF ascites are reported to represent

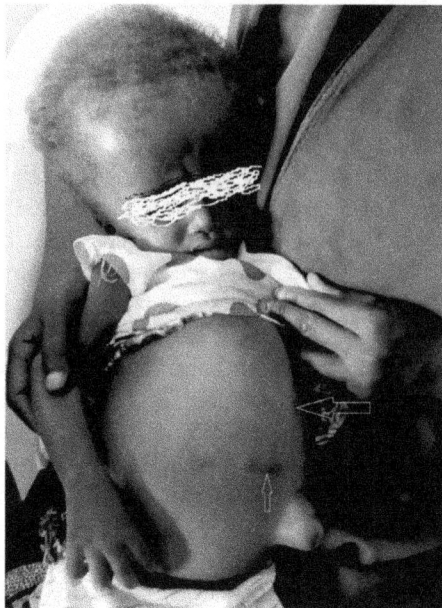

Figure 2.
A female child with severe shunt ascites, horizontal arrow showing shunt tubing and vertical arrow depicting abdominal scar.

5.8% of all VP shunt complications [10]. The proposed pathophysiological mechanisms of CSF ascites include: (1) elevation of CSF protein from infections or tumours leading to increasing intraperitoneal oncotic pressure and consequent CSF accumulation within the peritoneum. (2) Overwhelming CSF production from choroid plexus papilloma or carcinoma exceeding the absorptive capacity of the peritoneum. (3) Clinical or sub-clinical peritonitis impairing lymphatic absorption [10, 11] CSF ascites can be graded into 1 (mild, detectable only on ultrasound, CT or MRI of the abdomen), grade 2 or moderate (clinically detectable with bulging flanks and shifting dullness), and grade 3 or severe (easily visible, confirmed with fluid thrill, also called fluid wave test). Other common causes of ascites like liver disease, cardiac, renal, and malnutrition should be ruled out in patients with CSF ascites. A CSF sample should be sent for microbiological analysis and biochemistry as well as cytology in order to find out the possible cause of the condition. CSF diversion to other spaces such as pleura, cardiac, or even endoscopic third ventriculostomy allows resolution of ascites usually within 2 weeks (**Figure 2**).

12. Shunt calcification

Shunt calcification remains an uncommon complication of VP shunt; the first reported case was in 1988. The deposition of calcium and other minerals in addition to fibrosis led to shunt malfunction from either tube tethering and obstruction or disconnection. Calcification can occur in both metastatic and dystrophic forms. Patients with features of shunt calcification should have serum calcium evaluated, and require shunt revision, excision of calcified tissue entangling the shunt, and histological analysis [12].

13. Intraparenchymal/intraventricular haemorrhage

In the course of shunt insertion into the ventricles, meningeal, cerebral, or ventricular blood vessels may be injured, leading to intracerebral or intraventricular haemorrhages or both. Haemorrhages are usually mild in the absence of coagulopathy, requiring no specific treatment. Meticulous surgical technique, coagulation of meninges, and pre-operative evaluation of bleeding tendencies are paramount in preventing these complications. These haemorrhages may cause seizures, early shunt blockage (intraventricular), and early post-operative clinical deterioration. Primary haemorrhage noticed immediately after insertion of a ventricular catheter into the ventricle requires the surgeon to wait for a few minutes for clearance of the bleed, which usually stops except when coagulopathy exists, before connecting to the distal tubing. Massive or persistent haemorrhage may warrant externalisation of shunt tubing as external ventricular drainage.

14. Undershunting/overshunting

Shunt may malfunction, draining an amount of CSF below the volume required to keep intracranial pressure (ICP) within normal range. It may result from an abnormal or dysfunctional shunt valve; it may also result from partial shunt occlusion by proteinaceous debris, choroid plexus, or blood clot. Patients usually present with headache, increasing head size, vomiting, impaired vision, and other features of raised ICP. Overshunting occurs when the shunt valve becomes dysfunctional, draining much more CSF to the extent of causing intracranial hypotension and slit ventricle. Subdural haematomas may also result from overshunting. Ventriculoperitoneal shunt is more likely to be associated with overshunting than ventriculoatrial or pleural because of the high risk of siphoning effect [9]. Both undershunting and overshunting require shunt revision to allow proper CSF drainage and general well-being and health of the hydrocephalic patients.

15. Skull deformity

Skull deformities such as craniosynostosis or an abnormally shaped skull may occur in patients shunted for hydrocephalus. Deformities may result from rapid normalisation of intracranial pressure and collapse of the skull in infants and subsequent fusion in an abnormally shaped state. Sometimes poor nursing or parental care, such as keeping an infant shunted for hydrocephalus for a long time in one position, causes skull deformity. Deformity may be self-limiting, and disfiguring cases require cosmetic cranioplasty.

16. Seizure

Seizure is a known complication of VP shunt occurring in about 5.5%. It may result from initial cortical irritation and cerebral injury by the ventricular catheter. It may also be from intracerebral haemorrhage that may occur. It's reported that inserting a shunt via frontal points (Kocher's) has more risk of seizure compared to parieto-occipital points (keens). Patients developing seizures require anticonvulsants and a brain CT scan or MRI to ascertain the cause.

17. Silicon reactions

Pudenz made the first shunt made up of silicon in 1955 for treatment of hydrocephalus. Silicone (polysiloxanes) is one of the most commonly used inert materials in medicine. It has minimal biological reactivity, high flexibility, and chemical stability and is bound by fillers used and employed in the manufacturing of medical silicon. Biological reactivity of silicon is hypothesised to result from biological degradation of the implants, erosion of fillers, and exposure of antigen to body immune cells. Also, macrophage conversion of silicon to silica exposes antigens to the immune system, and silicon microparticles may act as haptens and thus cause immunological reactions. Chronic reactions to silicon include minimal inflammatory reaction, fibrous tissue formation, and pseudocapsule around the shunt tubing. Winer and Sternberg reported granuloma formation termed siliconomas [13]. Silicon reactions may resemble shunt infection with skin breakdown and fungating granulomas; csf initially sterile but may become infected and may require the creation of a customised silicon-free shunt like polyurethane.

18. CSF shunt as conduits for metastasis

CSF shunts have been reported to serve as conduits for dissemination of malignancy. The spread could be antegrade (extra-neural metastasis), where tumour cells from the brain are transported via shunt to the extra-neural part of the body, or retrograde metastasis, an event where tumour cells located elsewhere in the body dislodge and travel via CSF shunt and get deposited along the shunt tract up to the brain and ventricles. The most common brain tumours associated with extra-neural CSF shunt metastasis include germinomas (24.79%), medulloblastomas (18.18%), and glioblastomas (12.40%) [14–18]. Location of metastasis include peritoneum (85.95%), liver (14.88%), lymph node (14.05%), diaphragm (9.09%) and pleura (6.61%). Treatment of extra-neural antegrade metastasis includes radiotherapy, chemotherapy, and surgical excision.

Retrograde CSF shunt metastasis also occurs, with half of reported cases deposited along the shunt tract in cutaneous or subcutaneous tissues and the other half in the brain manifesting with neurological features [19–23]. Primary tumours originated in the abdomen or pelvis. Malignant tumours implicated in retrograde metastasis include pancreatic, ovarian, liver, gastrointestinal, gall bladder tumours, and colorectal tumours. The treatment for retrograde metastasis depends on the primary tumours, clinical status of the patient, and presence of cerebral metastasis. A CSF shunt is diverted to pleural or atrial; chemotherapy and radiotherapy will help in controlling tumour burden (**Tables 1** and **2**).

Primary brain tumours	Percentage metastasis
Germinoma	24.79
Medulloblastoma	18.18
Glioblastoma	12.40
Pineoblastoma	4.13
Ependymoma	2.48
Source: Refs. [15, 16].	

Table 1.
Primary brain tumours that metastasise.

Sites	Percentage metastasis
Peritoneum	85.95
Liver	14.88
Lymph nodes	14.05
Bone	12.40
Pleura	6.61
Source: Refs. [15, 16].	

Table 2.
Metastatic locations.

19. Shuntalgia

Is an uncommon complication of VP shunting characterised by discomfort and pain around the shunt tract. It results from focal inflammation and fibrosis around the shunt tubing. It is common amongst adolescents and requires counselling and optimal analgesia [15].

20. Conclusion

Complications of ventriculoperitoneal shunts are common and can occur in any part of the body along the pathway of the shunt tubing from the cranial to the peritoneal cavities. Optimal patient evaluation, meticulous surgical techniques, as well as careful patient's selection, will go a long way in preventing disability and death associated with ventriculoperitoneal shunt surgery.

Acknowledgements

We would like to appreciate the entire staff of neurosurgery department of Usmanu Danfodiyo University teaching Hospital Sokoto for their cooperation in management of hydrocephalic patients.

Conflict of interest

The Authors declare no conflict of interest.

Author details

Aliyu Muhammad Koko[1]* and Muhammad Mansur Idris[2]

1 Department of Surgery, Faculty of Clinical Sciences, College of Health Sciences, Usmanu Danfodiyo University Sokoto, Nigeria

2 Department of Neurosurgery, National Hospital Abuja, Abuja, FCT, Nigeria

*Address all correspondence to: aliyu.koko@udusok.edu.ng

IntechOpen

References

[1] Pa M et al. Ventriculoperitoneal shunt complications: A review. 2018;**13**(2017):66-70. DOI: 10.1016/j.inat.2018.04.004

[2] Merkler AE et al. HHS Public Access. 2018. pp. 654-658. DOI:10.1016/j.wneu.2016.10.136

[3] Reddy GK, Bollam P, Caldito G. Long term outcomes of ventriculoperitoneal shunt surgery in patients with hydrocephalus. World Neurosurgery. 2014;**81**(2):404-410. DOI: 10.1016/j.wneu.2013.01.096. Epub 2013 Feb 4

[4] McGirt MJ, Leveque J, Wellons JC, Villavicencio AT, Hopkins JS, Fuchs HE. Cerebrospinal fluid shunt survival and etiology of failures: A seven year institutional experience. Pediatric Neurosurgery. 2002;**36**:248-255

[5] Stone JJ, Walker CT, Jacobson M, Phillips V, Silberstein HJ. Revision rate of pediatric ventriculoperitoneal shunts after 15 years. Journal of Neurosurgery. Pediatrics. 2013;**11**:15-19

[6] Hasanain AA, Abdullah A, Alsawy MFM, Soliman MAR, Ghaleb AA, Elwy R, et al. Incidence of and causes for Ventriculoperitoneal shunt failure in children younger than 2 years: A systematic review. Journal of Neurological Surgery Part A: Central European Neurosurgery. 2019;**80**(1):26-33. DOI: 10.1055/s-0038-1669464. Epub 2018 Dec 3

[7] Moshref R, Algethmi RA. Systemic review: Neurological deficits following ventriculoperitoneal shunt (VPS) insertion. 2023;**18**(3):444-453. DOI: 10.1055/s-0043-1771329

[8] Chung J et al. Intraabdominal Complications Shunts: CT Findings and Review of the Literature (November).

2009. pp. 1311-1317. DOI:10.2214/AJR.09.2463

[9] Daibu U et al. Surgical Management and Outcomes of Childhood Hydrocephalus in a Resource-Challenged Setting in Northeast Nigeria (January). 2025. DOI: 10.46900/apn.v7i1.290

[10] Ferreira Furtado LM, Da Costa Val Filho JA, Moreira Faleiro R, Lima Vieira JA, Dantas Dos Santos AK. Abdominal complications related to ventriculoperitoneal shunt placement: A comprehensive review of literature. Cureus. 2021;**13**(2):e13230. DOI: 10.7759/cureus.13230

[11] Ayogu OM et al. World neurosurgery: X ventriculoperitoneal shunt infection rate and other associated complications of VP shunt insertion in Abuja, Nigeria. World Neurosurgery: X. 2024;**23**(January):100332. DOI: 10.1016/j.wnsx.2024.100332

[12] Harsh GR. Peritoneal shunt for hydrocephalus, utilizing the fimbria of the fallopian tube for entrance to the peritoneal cavity. Journal of Neurosurgery. 1954;**11**(3):284-294. DOI: 10.3171/jns.1954.11.3.0284

[13] Latchaw JPJ, Hahn JF. Intraperitoneal pseudocyst associated with peritoneal shunt. Neurosurgery. 1981;**8**(4):469-472. DOI: 10.1227/00006123-198104000-00013

[14] Rainov N et al. Abdominal CSF pseudocysts in patients with ventriculo-peritoneal shunts. Report of fourteen cases and review of the literature. Acta Neurochirurgica. 1994;**127**(1-2):73-78. DOI: 10.1007/BF01808551

[15] Hoffman HJ, Duffner PK. Extraneural metastases of central

nervous system tumors. Cancer. 1985;**56**(Suppl. 7):1778-1782

[16] Back MR, Hu B, Rutgers J, French S, Moore TC. Metastasis of an intracranial germinoma through a ventriculoperitoneal shunt: Recurrence as a yolk-sac tumor. Pediatric Surgery International. 1997;**12**(1):24-27

[17] Lam S et al. Management of hydrocephalus in children with posterior fossa tumors. Surgical Neurology International. 2015;**6**:S346-S348. DOI: 10.4103/2152-7806.161413

[18] Popa F et al. Laparoscopic treatment of abdominal complications following ventriculoperitoneal shunt. Journal of Medicine and Life. 2009;**2**(4):426-436

[19] Suleiman SE et al. Ventriculoperitoneal shunt-associated ascites: A case report. Cureus. 2020;**12**(6):1-9. DOI: 10.7759/cureus.8634

[20] Koko AM et al. Uncommon complications of ventriculoperitoneal shunt surgery: Review of four cases and literature review. Egyptian Journal of Neurosurgery. 2020;**35**(1):2-6. DOI: 10.1186/s41984-019-0071-6

[21] Jimenez DF, Keating R, Goodrich JT. Silicone allergy in ventriculoperitoneal shunts. Child's Nervous System. 1994;**10**(1):59-63. DOI: 10.1007/BF00313586

[22] Cuschieri A, Pisani R, Agius S. CSF shunts as conduits for metastasis: Is there a discrepancy between retrograde and antegrade spread? Egyptian Journal of Neurosurgery. 2025;**40**:37. DOI: 10.1186/s41984-025-00383-z

[23] Bauman N, Poenaru D. Hydrocephalus in Africa: A surgical perspective. Annals of African Surgery. 2008;**2**(September):30-37. DOI: 10.4314/aas.v2i1.46240

Chapter 5

Post-Traumatic Hydrocephalus: Diagnosis and Treatment

*Mattia Capobianco, Mauro Palmieri, Giuseppa Zancana,
Antonio Santoro and Alessandro Frati*

Abstract

Post-traumatic hydrocephalus (PTH) complicates very frequently the clinical course of patients with moderate to severe head injury (up to 20% of these patients). Nowadays, the pathogenesis of PTH is still not clear. Pathological changes of cerebrospinal fluid (CSF) resulting from trauma are the result of altered factors widely described in the literature, like CSF dinamics (secretion, absorption, circulation), osmotic pressure load of CSF, intracranial pressure changes (intracranial hemorrhages, cerebral contusions, brain edema), surgical treatments. The scope of this chapter is to clarify the state of the art of this topic, discussing pathogenesis, diagnostic criteria, treatment and possible prevention.

Keywords: post-traumatic hydrocephalus, traumatic brain injury, shunt surgery, computed tomography, magnetic resonance imaging

1. Introduction

Post-traumatic hydrocephalus (PTH) is a significant neurological complication that occurs following traumatic brain injury (TBI), typically defined as hydrocephalus neurologic symptoms in the setting of radiographic ventriculomegaly and a history of brain trauma [1–3]. Head trauma, caused by external forces acting on the head, is a major cause of disability and mortality worldwide [4–6]. The etiopathogenesis of PTH is not yet fully understood, but it is believed to be caused by obstacles in the secretion, absorption and circulation of cerebrospinal fluid (CSF) within the ventricular system [5]. In practical terms, PTH manifests as an abnormal accumulation of CSF, leading to ventriculomegaly, or enlargement of the cerebral ventricles, due to imbalances in the circulation and absorption of CSF [5]. Previous studies found several risk factors, like lower Glasgow Coma Scale (GCS) score at admission, higher age, intraventricular/subarachnoid hemorrhage (IVH/SAH), decompressive craniectomy (DC) and meningitis [7].

PTH can have a significant impact on the quality of life and prognosis of patients with TBI, increasing morbidity and mortality as compared to TBI patients who do not develop PTH [5, 8–10]. A thorough understanding of its definition, classification, diagnostic criteria, treatment, and assessment of post-treatment effects is essential for effective prevention and management [5]. This chapter aims to provide a general over-view of the state of the art of this pathology through a literature review about this topic.

2. Epidemiology

The incidence of symptomatic PTH varies widely, with reported ranges from 0.7% to 29% [11, 12]. However, when computed tomography (CT) criteria of ventriculo-megaly are used, the incidence can range from 30% to 86% [11]. This wide variation is attributable to differences in diagnostic criteria and classification [11]. In particular, following decompressive craniectomy (DC) for TBI, the rate of PTH is high, ranging from 12% to 36% [5, 13]. One study reported that 21% of patients required ventricu-loperitoneal shunting (VPS) after hemicraniectomy for severe TBI [13]. In an analysis of 500 cases of head trauma, the incidence of radiological PTH was found to be 3.4% [14]. The prevalence of PTH may change between different studied populations and relative to the criteria used for diagnosis. For example, a large retrospective study of 1941 adult patients with head trauma found that only 0.15% met the clinical and radio-logical diagnosis of PTH and benefited from a ventriculoperitoneal shunt [15, 16].

3. Etiology and pathophysiology

The precise etiology of PTH is not fully understood, but several mechanisms are thought to contribute to its development [5, 7, 13–15].

CSF flow obstruction: TBI can cause hemorrhage, edema, and inflammation, which can obstruct the CSF flow pathways, leading to the accumulation of CSF in the ventricles [5]. Obstruction may occur at the foramina of Monro, the aqueduct of Sylvius, or the foramina of Luschka and Magendie [17–19].

Decreased CSF absorption: CSF is reabsorbed mostly by the arachnoid villi at the Pacchioni granulations adjacent to the superior sagittal sinus. TBI may damage these villi, reducing the capacity for CSF absorption [5].

Increased cerebral venous pressure may also impair CSF drainage and contribute to ventriculomegaly [20–22]. Furthermore, accumulation of blood "debris" resulting from the evolution of a subarachnoid hemorrhage (SAH) or a hemoventricle may significantly slow CSF reabsorption at the reabsorption stations or by causing fibrosis of the arachnoid membranes [7, 20]. A large retrospective study in 2019 found that patients with SAH after TBI had approximate threefold risk of developing PTH com-pared to TBI patients without traumatic SAH [19]. Other researchers suggest that the presence of an interhemispheric hygroma may be an indicator of such disturbances in CSF circulation [2, 3, 23].

Increased CSF production: In rare cases, TBI may cause increased CSF production by the choroid plexuses, overloading the capacity of the absorptive system [5].

3.1 Risk factors

Numerous risk factors have been identified for PTH, as reported below.

Low Glasgow Coma Scale (GCS) score on admission: A low GCS score on admis-sion (GCS = 3–8) following TBI indicates a higher risk of PTH [7, 17, 18].

High Injury Severity Score (ISS): A higher ISS indicates greater overall injury severity, increasing the risk of PTH [13].

Presence of subarachnoid hemorrhage (SAH): As previously discussed, SAH is a significant risk factor for PTH [1, 7, 18–20, 24, 25].

Decompressive craniectomy (DC): DC, the surgical procedure of choice used to reduce intracranial pressure in severe TBI, is associated with an increased risk of PTH [7, 18]. Furthermore, studies have shown that younger patients undergoing DC are at increased risk of developing PTH [12, 13]. Regarding surgical technique, additional risk factors have been identified. Large cranial opercula and a medial limit of craniectomy <25 mm from the midline may increase the risk of PTH [13].

Delayed cranioplasty: Delay in repositioning of the cranial operculum after DC has been identified as a risk factor for PTH [1–3, 13, 23, 26–33]. In general, a >3 months cranioplasty has been associated with increased hazard for PTH [28].

Interhemispheric hygroma: The presence of an interhemispheric hygroma is associated with an increased risk of PTH [2, 3, 23].

Contralateral subdural hematoma: The presence of a subdural hematoma on the side opposite the DC has been identified as a risk factor [23, 34].

Prolonged ventilatory support: The need for prolonged mechanical ventilation is associated with an increased risk of PTH [14, 25].

Post-traumatic meningitis: Infection of the meninges following TBI (e.g., head trauma with open fractures or post-traumatic cerebrospinal fluid fistula) can cause meningeal inflammation and fibrosis, impeding CSF flow and absorption [35].

4. Classification

PTH can be classified based on several criteria [4, 5, 7, 12]: talking about the time of onset, and we can classify it as acute (develops within a few weeks after TBI), subacute (develops within a few weeks to a few months after TBI) and chronic PTH (develops several months or years after TBI). With respect to the physiopathological mechanism, PTH could be distinguished as communicating (the obstruction is outside the ventricular system, preventing reabsorption of CSF) and non-communicating or obstructive (the obstruction is within the ventricular system, blocking the flow of CSF). Regarding pressure, moreover, we can classify PTH as high pressure (characterized by elevated intracranial pressure) and normal pressure (characterized by normal intracranial pressure, but with ventriculomegaly and clinical symptoms) [4, 5, 7, 12].

5. Diagnosis

The diagnosis of PTH is based on a combination of clinical, imaging, and physiological findings [5, 7, 11, 12]. It can be difficult in patients with large craniotomy defects and abnormal post-traumatic anatomy [13]. It is important to distinguish PTH from ventriculomegaly "ex vacuo" (secondary to brain atrophy), especially in terms of treatment options [36–38].

5.1 Clinical assessment

Patients with PTH may present with a variety of symptoms, including headache, nausea, vomiting, lethargy, irritability and aggressiveness, gait disturbance, urinary incontinence, spasticity, recurrent epileptic seizures and cognitive decline [4, 5, 7, 11, 12, 15, 19]. In severe cases, patients may present with rapid neurologic deterioration, severe impairment of consciousness, or poor neurologic recovery [1, 5, 7, 11, 13, 15, 25]. Patients with ventriculomegaly "ex vacuo," in contrast, show stable neurologic deficits related to brain atrophy [20, 36–38]. It is important to note that symptoms may vary depending on the age of the patient, the severity of the TBI, and the time since the injury. Timing is important, as PTH typically develops a few weeks to several months after the injury [2, 4, 5, 7, 11–13, 17, 19, 24, 28].

5.2 Neuroimaging

Computed tomography (CT): CT is the most common initial imaging modality for evaluating PTH. It may reveal ventriculomegaly, cerebral edema, hemorrhages, and other structural abnormalities [5, 7, 11, 12, 23, 32, 39]. It is critical to distinguish symptomatic PTH from post-traumatic ventriculomegaly resulting from brain atrophy [20, 32, 39]. In the latter case, ventricular enlargement is due to loss of brain tissue, rather than active accumulation of CSF. The Evans index (>0.3), modified frontal horn index (mFHI >0.33), narrowed CSF spaces at the convexity, third ventricular enlargement, sharpening of the callosal angle and periventricular lucencies can be used to estimate the degree of ventricular dilation [1, 3, 36–38, 40]. However, these indices may not be reliable in patients who have undergone unilateral craniectomy [32]. Some authors suggest that temporal horn enlargement detects hydrocephalus earlier and faster than Evans index change [15].

Magnetic resonance imaging (MRI): MRI is more sensitive than CT for detecting small abnormalities and can provide more detailed information on CSF flow or kinetics and the patency of drainage pathways (e.g., assessment of CSF flow through the aqueduct of Sylvius defining absolute stroke volume and peak flow velocity) [5, 7, 11, 12, 32, 41–43].

5.3 Additional tests

Intracranial pressure (ICP) monitoring: ICP monitoring may be useful in identifying patients with high-pressure hydrocephalus. However, it is not always necessary for the diagnosis of PTH, particularly in cases of normal-pressure hydrocephalus [5, 11–14].

Lumbar puncture: A lumbar puncture can measure the CSF opening pressure and analyze the CSF contents. This can help distinguish between hydrocephalus and other conditions, such as meningitis [6]. Furthermore, the removal of 30–50 ml of CSF (Tap Test AKA Miller Fisher test) is useful for the selection of those patients who may benefit from shunting [5, 11–14].

CSF dynamics tests: Infusion tests can be used to evaluate CSF outflow resistance or impedance (Ro) and intracranial pressure [36–38]. Marmarou et al. suggested differentiating ventriculomegaly "ex vacuo" from post-traumatic hydrocephalus using such tests [36]. Patients with PTH may show greater CSF outflow resistance than those with hydrocephalus ex vacuo [20, 36–38]. Intracranial elastance and Ro may also help predict shunt responsiveness [20, 36–38].

6. Treatment

The primary goal of PTH treatment is to restore normal CSF flow and absorption, alleviating symptoms, normalizing intracranial pressure and preventing further neurological damage [5, 7, 11, 12, 27, 44, 45]. The choice of treatment depends on several factors, including the type and severity of PTH, the age and clinical condition of the patient, and the surgeon's preference (**Figure 1**).

Factors predisposing to surgical treatment are several, as reported below.

Symptomatic post-traumatic ventriculomegaly: Patients with symptomatic PTH are more likely to improve with surgical treatment, while ventriculomegaly secondary to atrophy ("ex vacuo") is less likely to respond to it [5, 7, 11–13, 36–38].

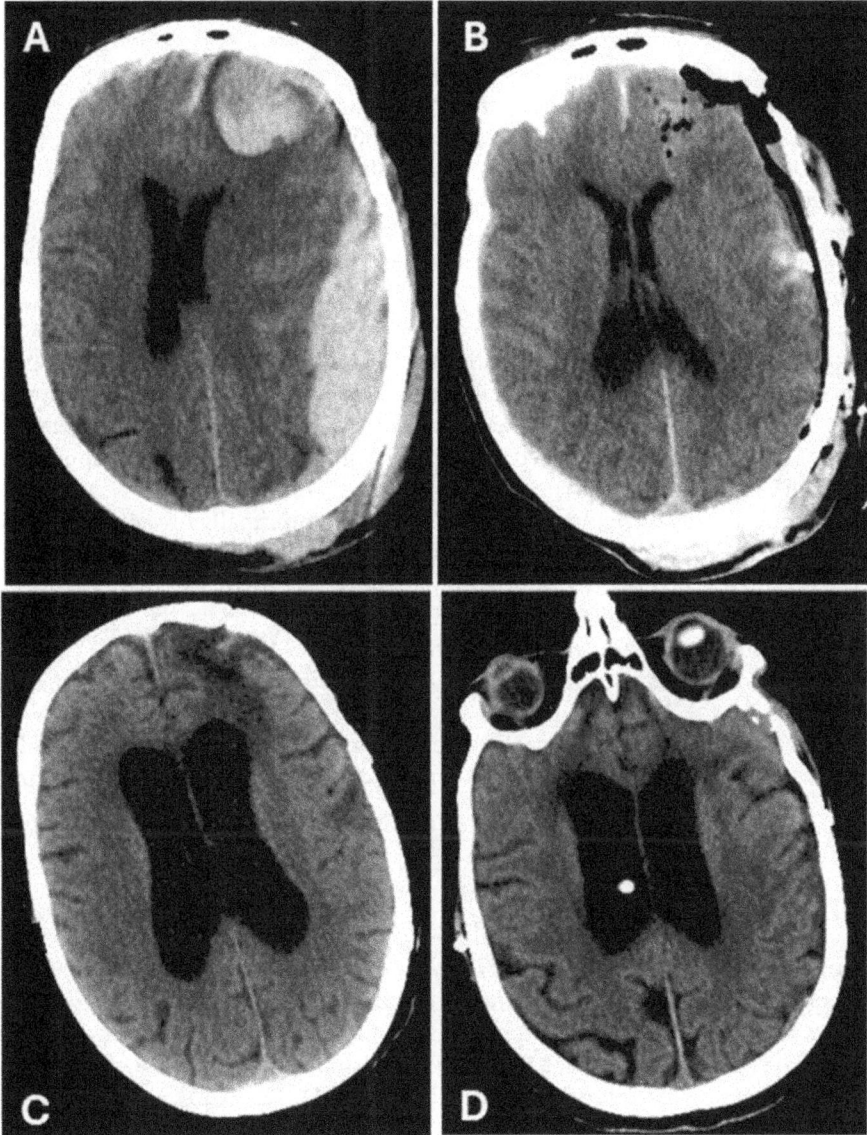

Figure 1.
CT images from a single severe TBI of 66 years old woman. A is a representative CT image during admission to hospital, which shows an acute left subdural/extradural hematoma and a left frontal lobe hematoma. B is a representative CT images of the patient from the immediate post-surgery period, which shows normal ventricular dimensions. C is a CT image 2 months after the injury. The patient, after initial neurological improvement, showed arrested functional recovery. The scan shows progressive PTH with transependymal reabsorption. D is a representative CT image during post-shunting period (3 months after TBI). The patient, after shunt surgery, showed total motor recovery, but maintained global aphasia.

Among symptoms, worsening neurological status, impaired consciousness, or poor neurological recovery are the most significant clinical factors for indicating surgical treatment [4, 5, 7, 11–13, 15].

Radiological findings showing progressive CSF accumulation, like ventricular dilation or a pattern of transependymal resorption, alteration of ventriculometric parameters (Evans, mFHI, temporal horns), narrowed CSF spaces at the convexity, third ventricular enlargement, sharpening of the callosal angle, MRI CSF kinetics alterations [5, 7, 13, 32, 39–43].

Increased intracranial pressure (ICP): CSF shunt procedures improve cases of ventriculomegaly with documented evidence of elevated ICP [13, 19, 28, 36–38, 44].

Symptoms of normal-pressure hydrocephalus: gait disturbances, urinary incontinence, and cognitive decline [5, 7, 11, 12, 15, 20, 36–38]. Patients with normal-pressure hydrocephalus have the best response to shunting [5, 7, 11, 12, 25, 29, 31, 36–38].

Papilledema [5, 7, 11–13].

Responsiveness to CSF dynamics tests [36–38].

Surgical treatment options include several techniques.

Ventriculoperitoneal shunt (VPS): VPS is the most common surgical procedure for PTH [5, 7, 11, 12, 19, 28, 29, 44]. In patients in whom peritoneal shunting is contraindicated, a ventriculoatrial shunt (VAS) may be a valid alternative [5, 7, 11]. Several studies have reported clinical improvements (as evaluated with various functional scales), in 52–78% of the patients after shunt surgery in PTH [46–48]. It is very important to improve patient selection due to common shunt surgery complications (almost 30% require shunt revision) [7].

Endoscopic third ventriculostomy (ETV): ETV is a minimally invasive surgical procedure that allows CSF to drain from the third ventricle directly into the subarachnoid spaces. ETV may be an effective option for patients with obstructive hydrocephalus, but is generally contraindicated in cases of PTH [45].

Cranioplasty: Early skull reconstruction after DC (<3 months after TBI) has been shown to improve cerebral perfusion and CSF dynamics, reducing the incidence of PTH [1, 2, 13, 26–28, 31, 33].

External lumbar drainage: In cases of acute communicating PTH, an external lumbar drain can be used temporarily to remove excess CSF and reduce intracranial pressure [7, 11, 12].

7. Prognosis

The prognosis for patients with PTH varies depending on several factors, including the underlying cause, severity and duration of hydrocephalus, and the timeliness of treatment [5, 7, 11, 12, 25]. Early diagnosis and shunt placement may improve long-term neurological recovery [4, 5, 7, 11, 12, 25, 32]. Some studies suggest that early shunting may lead to favorable outcomes during rehabilitation [11, 12, 19, 25]. However, the efficacy of CSF shunting for the treatment of PTH is not always supported by strong evidence [5, 7]. In some cases, post-traumatic damage may be too severe and result in a poor outcome [19, 28, 44]. Patients with symptoms of low-pressure hydrocephalus have demonstrated the best response to shunting, while those in a vegetative state have a minimal response [5, 7, 11, 12, 19]. PTH can lead to prolonged hospital stays and poor outcomes, especially if left untreated. In fact, PTH, if unrecognized and untreated, may have a significant impact on morbidity after TBI and may cause impaired neurologic recovery and increased mortality [5, 7, 11–13, 15, 19, 25, 29, 30].

8. Post-traumatic hydrocephalus in children

PTH in children presents unique challenges due to the growth and development of the brain [18, 49, 50]. Risk factors, treatment options, and outcomes may differ from adults. Younger children (0–5 years) had a higher risk of developing hydrocephalus compared to older age groups and certain type of injuries (open injuries, subdural hemorrhage, subarachnoid hemorrhage, shaken baby syndrome) are linked to higher rates of PTH [18, 49, 50]. Demographic, hospital, and clinical risk factors are associated with hydrocephalus development after TBI in children. Recognizing these factors can improve awareness and potentially reduce the incidence of PTH in this population [18, 49, 50].

9. Prevention

Prevention of PTH is critical to improving outcomes in patients with TBI. Preventive strategies may include several aspects.

Optimal management of acute TBI: Careful initial management of TBI, including control of intracranial pressure and prevention of complications, may reduce the risk of PTH [13, 44].

Early monitoring and intervention: Careful monitoring of TBI patients for signs and symptoms of PTH and early intervention when necessary may improve outcomes [32, 39, 44].

Judicious decompressive craniectomy: DC should be performed only when absolutely necessary and the surgical technique should be optimized to minimize the risk of PTH [1, 2, 27–31].

Timely cranioplasty: Timely skull closure after DC (<3 months) may help restore normal CSF dynamics and reduce the risk of PTH [1, 2, 23, 28–31].

10. Conclusion

Post-traumatic hydrocephalus is a complex and potentially devastating complication of TBI. Understanding its epidemiology, etiology, pathophysiology, risk factors, classification, diagnosis, treatment, and prognosis is essential for effective management of TBI. Early diagnosis, appropriate intervention, and preventive strategies can improve outcomes for patients with PTH. Future studies should focus on refining diagnostic classifications and criteria for PTH. Analysis of large PTH populations may help identify modifiable risk factors early in TBI, minimizing subsequent PTH and the need for shunts. Research should also focus on developing new therapies and management approaches to improve outcomes for patients with PTH.

Acknowledgements

The authors gratefully acknowledge the assistance of the Human Neurosciences Department (Neurosurgery Division) of "Sapienza" University in the preparation of this manuscript.

Conflict of interest

The authors have no relevant affiliations or financial involvement with any organization or entity with a financial interest in or financial conflict with the subject matter or materials discussed in the manuscript. This includes employment, consultancies, honoraria, stock ownership or options, expert testimony, grants or patents received or pending, or royalties.

Acronyms and abbreviations

PTH	post-traumatic hydrocephalus
CSF	cerebrospinal fluid
TBI	traumatic brain injury
DC	decompressive craniectomy
SAH	subarachnoid hemorrhage
GCS	Glasgow Coma Scale
CT	computed tomography
MRI	magnetic resonance imaging
mFHI	modified frontal horn index
ICP	intracranial pressure
VPS	ventriculoperitoneal shunt
VAS	ventriculoatrial shunt
ETV	endoscopic third ventriculostomy

Author details

Mattia Capobianco[1]*, Mauro Palmieri[1], Giuseppa Zancana[1], Antonio Santoro[1] and Alessandro Frati[1,2]

1 Human Neurosciences Department, Neurosurgery Division "Sapienza" University, Rome, Italy

2 IRCCS "Neuromed", Pozzilli (IS), Italy

*Address all correspondence to: mattia.capobianco@uniroma1.it

IntechOpen

References

[1] Honeybul S, Ho KM. Incidence and risk factors for post-traumatic hydrocephalus following decompressive craniectomy for intractable intracranial hypertension and evacuation of mass lesions. Journal of Neurotrauma. 2012;**29**(10):1872-1878

[2] De Bonis P, Sturiale CL, Anile C, Gaudino S, Mangiola A, Martucci M, et al. Decompressive craniectomy, interhemispheric hygroma and hydrocephalus: A timeline of events? Clinical Neurology and Neurosurgery. 2013;**115**(8):1308-1312

[3] Kaen A, Jimenez-Roldan L, Alday R, Gomez PA, Lagares A, Alén JF, et al. Interhemispheric hygroma after decompressive craniectomy: Does it predict posttraumatic hydrocephalus? Journal of Neurosurgery. 2010;**113**(6):1287-1293

[4] De Bonis P, Anile C. Post-traumatic hydrocephalus: The cinderella of neurotrauma. Expert Review of Neurotherapeutics. 2020;**20**(7):643-646

[5] Li Z, Zhang H, Hu G, Zhang G. Post-traumatic hydrocephalus: An overview of classification, diagnosis, treatment, and post-treatment imaging evaluation. Brain Research Bulletin. 2023;**205**:110824

[6] Brazinova A, Rehorcikova V, Taylor MS, Buckova V, Majdan M, Psota M, et al. Epidemiology of traumatic brain injury in Europe: A living systematic review. Journal of Neurotrauma. 2021;**38**(10):1411-1440

[7] Svedung Wettervik T, Lewén A, Enblad P. Post-traumatic hydrocephalus—Incidence, risk factors, treatment, and clinical outcome. British Journal of Neurosurgery. 2022;**36**(3):400-406

[8] Sun S, Zhou H, Ding ZZ, Shi H. Risk factors associated with the outcome of post-traumatic hydrocephalus. Scandinavian Journal of Surgery. 2019;**108**(3):265-270

[9] Huh PW, Yoo DS, Cho KS, Park CK, Kang SG, Park YS, et al. Diagnostic method for differentiating external hydrocephalus from simple subdural hygroma. Journal of Neurosurgery. 2006;**105**(1):65-70

[10] Beaumont A, Marmarou A. Treatment of raised intracranial pressure following traumatic brain injury. Critical Reviews in Neurosurgery. 1999;**9**(4):207-216

[11] Guyot LL, Michael DB. Post-traumatic hydrocephalus. Neurological Research. 2000;**22**(1):25-28

[12] Rufus P, Moorthy RK, Joseph M, Rajshekhar V. Post traumatic hydrocephalus. Neurology India. 2021;**69**(Suppl 2):S420-S428

[13] Goldschmidt E, Deng H, Puccio AM, Okonkwo DO. Post-traumatic hydrocephalus following decompressive hemicraniectomy: Incidence and risk factors in a prospective cohort of severe TBI patients. Journal of Clinical Neuroscience. 2020;**73**:85-88

[14] Jha VC, Jha N. Post Traumatic Hydrocephalus in Indian Subpopulation: An Institutional Experience. Turkish Neurosurgery. 2023;**33**(1):10-17

[15] Missori P, Paolini S, Currà A. Prevalence of post-traumatic hydrocephalus in moderate to severe head injury. Acta Neurochirurgica. 2022;**165**(2):299-300

[16] Heinonen A, Rauhala M, Isokuortti H, Kataja A, Nikula M, Öhman J, et al. Incidence of surgically treated post-traumatic hydrocephalus 6 months following head injury in patients undergoing acute head computed tomography. Acta Neurochirurgica. 2022;**164**(9):2357-2365

[17] Shah AH, Komotar RJ. Pathophysiology of acute hydrocephalus after subarachnoid hemorrhage. World Neurosurgery. 2013;**80**(3-4):304-306

[18] Spennato P, Ruggiero C, Parlato RS, Trischitta V, Mirone G, De Santi MS, et al. Acute post-traumatic hydrocephalus in children due to aqueductal obstruction by blood clot: A series of 6 patients. Child's Nervous System. 2019;**35**(11):2037-2041

[19] Chen KH, Lee CP, Yang YH, Yang YH, Chen CM, Lu ML, et al. Incidence of hydrocephalus in traumatic brain injury. Medicine. 2019;**98**(42):e17568

[20] Aso T, Sugihara G, Murai T, Ubukata S, Urayama S-I, Ueno T, et al. A venous mechanism of ventriculomegaly shared between traumatic brain injury and normal ageing. Brain. 2020;**143**(6):1843-1856

[21] Zhao J, Chen Z, Xi G, Keep RF, Hua Y. Deferoxamine attenuates acute hydrocephalus after traumatic brain injury in rats. Translational Stroke Research. 2014;**5**(5):586-594

[22] Makinde HM, Just TB, Cuda CM, Bertolino N, Procissi D, Schwulst SJ. Monocyte depletion attenuates the development of posttraumatic hydrocephalus and preserves white matter integrity after traumatic brain injury. PLoS ONE. 2018;**13**(11):e0202722

[23] Lu VM, Carlstrom LP, Perry A, Graffeo CS, Domingo RA, Young CC, et al. Prognostic significance of subdural hygroma for post-traumatic hydrocephalus after decompressive craniectomy in the traumatic brain injury setting: A systematic review and meta-analysis. Neurosurgical Review. 2021;**44**(1):129-138

[24] Tian HL, Xu T, Hu J, Cui Y-h, Chen H, Zhou LF. Risk factors related to hydrocephalus after traumatic subarachnoid hemorrhage. Surgical Neurology. 2008;**69**(3):241-246

[25] Linnemann M, Tibæk M, Kammersgaard LP. Hydrocephalus during rehabilitation following severe TBI. Relation to recovery, outcome, and length of stay. NeuroRehabilitation. 2014;**35**(4):755-761

[26] Waziri A, Fusco D, Mayer SA, McKhann GM, Connolly ES. Postoperative hydrocephalus in patients undergoing decompressive hemicraniectomy for ischemic or hemorrhagic stroke. Neurosurgery. 2007;**61**(3):489-494

[27] Sahuquillo J, Dennis JA. Decompressive craniectomy for the treatment of high intracranial pressure in closed traumatic brain injury. Cochrane Database of Systematic Reviews. 2019 Dec 31;**12**(12):CD003983

[28] Nasi D, Gladi M, Di Rienzo A, di Somma L, Moriconi E, Iacoangeli M, et al. Risk factors for post-traumatic hydrocephalus following decompressive craniectomy. Acta Neurochirurgica. 2018;**160**(9):1691-1698

[29] Missori P, Currà A, Peschillo S, Paolini S. Post-traumatic hydrocephalus after decompressive craniectomy. Journal of Clinical Neuroscience. 2021;**93**:268-269

[30] Cooper DJ, Rosenfeld JV, Murray L, Arabi YM, Davies AR, D'Urso P, et al. Decompressive craniectomy in diffuse traumatic brain injury. New England Journal of Medicine. 2011;**364**(16):1493-1502

[31] Vedantam A, Yamal JM, Hwang H, Robertson CS, Gopinath SP. Factors associated with shunt-dependent hydrocephalus after decompressive craniectomy for traumatic brain injury. Journal of Neurosurgery. 2018;**128**(5):1547-1552

[32] Huang YH, Lee TH. Characteristics of post-traumatic shunt-dependent hydrocephalus after decompressive craniectomy: Are computed tomography scoring systems predictors? World Neurosurgery. 2024;**190**:e263-e270

[33] Williams JR, Meyer RM, Ricard JA, Sen R, Young CC, Feroze AH, et al. Re-examining decompressive craniectomy medial margin distance from midline as a metric for calculating the risk of post-traumatic hydrocephalus. Journal of Clinical Neuroscience. 2021;**87**:125-131

[34] Haines DE, Harkey HL, Al-Mefty O. The "Subdural" space. Neurosurgery. 1993;**32**(1):111-120

[35] Baltas I, Tsoulfa S, Sakellariou P, Vogas V, Fylaktakis M, Kondodimou A. Posttraumatic meningitis. Neurosurgery. 1994;**35**(3):422-427

[36] Marmarou A, Abd-Elfattah Foda MA, Bandoh K, Yoshihara M, Yamamoto T, Tsuji O, et al. Posttraumatic ventriculomegaly: Hydrocephalus or atrophy? A new approach for diagnosis using CSF dynamics. Journal of Neurosurgery. 1996;**85**(6):1026-1035

[37] De Bonis P, Mangiola A, Pompucci A, Formisano R, Mattogno P, Anile C.

CSF dynamics analysis in patients with post-traumatic ventriculomegaly. Clinical Neurology and Neurosurgery. 2013;**115**(1):49-53

[38] Lalou AD, Levrini V, Czosnyka M, Gergelé L, Garnett M, Kolias A, et al. Cerebrospinal fluid dynamics in non-acute post-traumatic ventriculomegaly. Fluids and Barriers of the CNS. 2020;**17**(1):24

[39] Gudeman SK, Kishore PR, Becker DP, Lipper MH, Girevendulis AK, Jeffries BF, et al. Computed tomography in the evaluation of incidence and significance of post-traumatic hydrocephalus. Radiology. 1981;**141**(2):397-402

[40] Pyrgelis ES, Paraskevas GP, Constantinides VC, Boufidou F, Velonakis G, Stefanis L, et al. Callosal angle sub-score of the radscale in patients with idiopathic normal pressure hydrocephalus is associated with positive tap test response. Journal of Clinical Medicine. 2022;**11**(10):2898

[41] Govindarajan B, Sharma PK, Polaka Y, Pujitha S, Natarajan P. The role of phase-contrast MRI in diagnosing cerebrospinal fluid flow abnormalities. Cureus. 2024

[42] Chen CH, Cheng YC, Huang CY, Chen HC, Chen WH, Chai JW. Accuracy of MRI derived cerebral aqueduct flow parameters in the diagnosis of idiopathic normal pressure hydrocephalus. Journal of Clinical Neuroscience. 2022;**105**:9-15

[43] Ahmad N, Salama D, Al-Haggar M. MRI CSF flowmetry in evaluation of different neurological diseases. Egyptian Journal of Radiology and Nuclear Medicine. 2021;**52**(1):53

[44] Carney N, Totten AM, O'Reilly C, Ullman JS, Hawryluk GWJ, Bell MJ, et al.

Guidelines for the management of severe traumatic brain injury, fourth edition. Neurosurgery. 2017;**80**(1):6-15

[45] De Bonis P, Tamburrini G, Mangiola A, Pompucci A, Mattogno PP, Porso M, et al. Post-traumatic hydrocephalus is a contraindication for endoscopic third-ventriculostomy: Is n't it? Clinical Neurology and Neurosurgery. 2013;**115**(1):9-12

[46] Wen L, Wan S, Zhan RY, Li G, Gong JB, Liu WG, et al. Shunt implantation in a special sub-group of post-traumatic hydrocephalus—Patients have normal intracranial pressure without clinical representations of hydrocephalus. Brain Injury. 2009;**23**(1):61-64

[47] Oder GTW. Outcome after shunt implantation in severe head injury with post-traumatic hydrocephalus. Brain Injury. 2000;**14**(4):345-354

[48] Denes Z, Barsi P, Szel I, Boros E, Fazekas G. Complication during postacute rehabilitation. International Journal of Rehabilitation Research. 2011;**34**(3):222-226

[49] Elsamadicy AA, Koo AB, Lee V, David WB, Zogg CK, Kundishora AJ, et al. Risk factors for the development of post-traumatic hydrocephalus in children. World Neurosurgery. 2020;**141**:e105-e111

[50] Bonow RH, Oron AP, Hanak BW, Browd SR, Chesnut RM, Ellenbogen RG, et al. Post-traumatic hydrocephalus in children: A retrospective study in 42 pediatric hospitals using the pediatric health information system. Neurosurgery. 2018;**83**(4):732-739

Chapter 6

Alternative Methods in the Surgical Treatment of Hydrocephalus

Valentin Titus Grigorean and Alexandru Vlad Ciurea

Abstract

Hydrocephalus is a condition with a major impact on the noble cerebral substance, which, in the absence of a rapid and effective solution, generates significant morbidity and mortality. It is an eminently surgical pathology. The surgical solutions imagined are very numerous: ventriculo-cisternostomies, ventriculoperitoneal shunts, ventriculocardiac shunts, ventriculopleural shunts, ventriculobiliary shunts, ventriculovesical shunts, lumboperitoneal shunts, etc., with broader or narrower indications, sometimes with complications that can limit/restrict the procedure, requiring successive revisions or replacement of the method. Testing the viability and durability of each method imagined has been a constant concern during decades of neurosurgical practice. The occurrence of limited efficacy or complications recorded for each method in particular has generated attempts to improve and optimise the surgical technique, successive revisions of the method, or the choice of another surgical technique. The test of time has confirmed that the ventriculoperitoneal and ventriculocardiac shunts are the most viable and indicated in most etiopathogenic entities of hydrocephalus. This aspect has not limited the concerns for finding alternative surgical treatment solutions for situations in which their efficacy is exceeded or compromised. Ventriculoepiploic shunt, transomphalic extraperitoneal ventriculoportal shunt, and right transcephalic ventriculosubclavicular/ventriculocaval/ventriculocardiac shunt are innovative methods that may represent backup solutions in case of therapeutic failure.

Keywords: shunt, hydrocephalus, ventriculoperitoneal, ventriculosubclavicular, ventriculoepiploic

1. Introduction

Hydrocephalus is a multifactorial disease that consists in the accumulation of excess cerebrospinal fluid in an unextensible space to the detriment of the noble nerve substance. It can occur at any age, being discovered even intrauterine, and can settle in 8–9 decades of life. Of course, the aetiology is different; it can represent the epiphenomenon of a multitude of primitive conditions or the cause cannot be identified with certainty (cryptogenetic hydrocephalus), and the clinical manifestations can be different depending on a number of parameters: age, aetiology, pressure of the cerebrospinal fluid, etc.

Early diagnosis and the establishment of appropriate therapeutic measures are essential conditions for achieving the best possible postoperative results [1].

IntechOpen

2. Surgical treatment of hydrocephalus

2.1 Surgical treatment

It's based on the following surgical solutions:

- Treatment of the cause (surgery of malformations of the central nervous system, tumours of various structures that disrupt the physiological circulation of the cerebrospinal fluid, optimal resolution of post-traumatic brain injuries, etc.). This desire is not always possible and does not guarantee the immediate resolution of hydrocephalus that may assume a residual or recurrent character [2].

- Intersectoral redistribution of excess cerebrospinal fluid. Thus, ventriculostomy III realises the communication between the dilated ventricular system upstream and the subarachnoid interpeduncular cistern by perforating the floor of the ventricle III. The procedure is endoscopic and is reserved for obstructive hydrocephalus in patients with normal cerebrospinal fluid. Apeductoplasty (mounting of stents at the Sylvius aqueduct) may be associated. The technique is minimally invasive, involves low risks, and has superior efficiency if the surgical indication and technique are correct [3].

- External drainage involves the installation of a ventricular catheter that drains cerebrospinal fluid into an external tank. It is a "damage" solution and is limited in time (risk of ventricular contamination with consecutive meningitis). It is also accompanied by hydroelectrolytic and protein imbalances, which must be corrected promptly. It is indicated in case of meningitis-associated hydrocephalus or intraventricular haemorrhage, in case of shunt infection, transient hydrocephalus, or in the absence of a temporary surgical solution.

- Extracranial drainage involves communication between the dilated ventricular system and a preformed internal cavity or structure capable of taking in excess cerebrospinal fluid in a physiological way.

Communication is carried out through a dedicated piping and is conditioned by a number of factors:

- Pressure gradient between the ventricular system and the receiving cavity/structure

- Good tolerance of the cerebrospinal fluid in the structure that receives the cerebrospinal fluid

- Increased ability to absorb/take up excess cerebrospinal fluid

- Sterile receptor environment to avoid retrograde infections

- Walk as short as possible straight to avoid tubing bends that can cause flow dysfunctions

- Suitable silastic tubing and self-regulating pressure valves to avoid overdrainage phenomenons that can cause complications at the brain level (cerebroventricular collapse, subdural hematomas, chronic subdural hygroamas, ventricular slit syndrome, post-shunt craniostenosis, pneumocephalia, etc.) [4].

Identifying an ideal surgical treatment option for hydrocephaly is a constant concern spanning decades of research, experimental studies, and surgical applications. Given the etiological polymorphism of hydrocephalus of particular individual characteristics and the possible limitations and contraindications of some proposed procedures, it was impossible to identify a single general solution valid in all cases.

Of the proposed methods, some had limited efficacy over time; others were plagued by inconveniences or complications of the most varied, restricting their use in medical practice.

Another category is represented by effective technical variants, which solve the problem of hydrocephaly in the long term with good clinical and imaging results but which, in certain circumstances (some known, others obscure), may lose their effectiveness by the appearance of inconveniences or complications that may temporarily or permanently compromise the adopted surgical solution. In such situations, long-term or temporary therapeutic alternatives are needed until the premises to return to the original variant are created.

The specialised literature records a multitude of technical variants (some with historical importance today), which tried to solve the problem of hydrocephalus as effectively as possible. They fit into two major categories of surgical techniques:

- Use of a different receiving structure than previously used

- The use of the same receiving structures, but changing the first path or using certain technical artefacts aimed at limiting the inconveniences or complications of the established procedure.

The conditions to be met by the receiving structure are as follows:

- High capacity of resorption/absorption of excess cerebrospinal fluid

- Good tolerance to the chemical composition of the cerebrospinal fluid and drainage tubing

- Rigorous sterility conditions

- Durability over time of the assembly that uses the respective anatomical structure

The above conditions are met by seroses with high resorptive capacity and vascular (venous) structures with high blood flow or related to such structures.

2.1.1 The ventriculoperitoneal shunt

It involves draining the dilated right lateral ventricle with the help of dedicated tubing with pressure valves, into the peritoneal cavity, tunneling subcutaneously to the edge of the costal rim, or right paraumbilical, where the slope is introduced into the peritoneum. The ventriculoperitoneal shunt is well tolerated and can be a long-lasting solution, but it can also cause a number of dysfunctions and complications. Dysfunctions of the proximal or intermediate segment of the assembly may be recorded (obstruction of the ventricular end of the catheter, hip infection, disconnection of the device, etc.), but the most common complications where related to the distal pole (catheter migration, pseudocysts of the cerebrospinal fluid, ascites of the cerebrospinal fluid, perforations of the intraperitoneal organs, intestinal occlusion, inguinal hernia, hydrocel, inflammatory processes of the intraperitoneal organs, etc.), the final consequence being the limitation or the stop of the resorption of the cerebrospinal fluid reached in the peritoneum as well as the appearance of complications, that require the suppression of this drainage path and the choice of another technical variant. The ventriculoperitoneal shunt is well tolerated, indicating a wide range of etiological circumstances of hydrocephalus. Sometimes, identifiable factors or unclear pathogenic elements can lead to the compromise of this drainage pathway, requiring shunt revisions, sometimes repetitive, or the choice of another temporary or definitive therapeutic solution. It represents the lasting solution for a significant percentage of cases of hydrocephalus, with a very different determinism [5].

2.1.2 The ventriculocardiac shunt

It's an alternative to the ventriculoperitoneal shunt, rarely being the first option. It benefits from the immense advantage of free uptake of large amounts of cerebrospinal fluid in a huge vascular bed (VCS, right atrium), where it is well tolerated. The installation of the proximal catheter presents no peculiarities, and the distal end should be located in the upper cavity system or in the right atrium. This aspect generates the need for periodic stretching, if the patient is a paediatric one (depending on the process of growth). Evaluation of this parameter can be done fluoroscopically periodically, since the short distal end involves the risk of catheter thrombosis, while a long distal end can have cardiac repercussions (often rebel arrhythmias on a specific treatment).

Surgical technique is standardised, consisting in the identification of the internal jugular vein at the level of the tributary, represented by the facial vein that is bound and cut. Through a limited venotomy, the distal end of the catheter is inserted, which is introduced through the bonnet of the facial vein into the jugular vein and led up to the level of the right atrium. Confirmation of the presence of the distal end of the catheter in the right atrium can be done by native or contrast fluoroscopy, catheter pressure measurement, transesophageal echocardiography, or electrocardiography (the appearance of a biphasic "p" wave after injection on the 3% saline catheter). Insertion of the distal end of the catheter can also be done percussively [6].

Unfortunately, the procedure is plagued by a significant number of various complications:

1. Intraoperative: rupture and the loss of the catheter in the superior cavity axis, gas embolism, severe rhythm disorders, valvular or cord lesions

2. Postoperative:

   - Fast complications: mechanical and infectious ('spinal nephritis'), as well as proximal complications (sub- and extra-dural hematomas, obstruction of the catheter with brain tissue, etc.)

- Late complications: catheter dysfunction, blocking of the catheter at the myocardial level, venous thrombosis, disconnection with catheter migration etc.

2.1.3 Lomboperitoneal shunt

It's indicated in non-communicating hydrocephaly with undilated ventricles. The procedure performs communication between the lumbar cistern and the peritoneal cavity [7].

The applicability of this method is quite limited, and the complications (arachnoiditis, radiculopathies, etc.) are relatively common.

2.1.4 The ventriculopleural shunt

It involves the drainage of the cerebrospinal fluid into the pleural cavity through a skin incision in the 2–5 intercostal spaces, dilatation of the muscles, and then the distal end of the tubing is located down into the pleural cavity. Functionality is limited over time, and secondary pleurisies are common [8].

2.1.5 Other techniques

Other techniques used are ventriculocholecystic shunt, ventriculoureteral shunt, ventriculomastoidian shunt, and thoracic canal drainage. These techniques have historic value, being met by numerous complications and early dysfunction.

Extensive studies and extensive meta-analysis have concluded that the first surgical treatment option in most cases of hydrocephaly is the ventriculoperitoneal shunt, followed by the ventriculocardiac shunt. Well tolerated and with increased efficiency, the two methods lead detached in the list of surgical procedures that ensure a definitive, or long-lasting, surgical solution.

Although the complication rates for both surgical techniques are not high, when they are found, it requires prompt medical-surgical management adapted to the type of complication that was found.

Shunt revisions (sometimes necessary) may use the same receiving structure or another and may be repetitive.

The identification of surgical treatment alternatives has always been a constant concern and is reserved for situations in which the established methods have become inoperative and relate in particular to the complications of the distal pole of the assembly or general order complications.

Alternative methods of surgical treatment in hydrocephalus can use the same receiving structure (or derived from it), with technical artefacts of the location of the drainage tubing (to limit the inconveniences that were at the basis of the appearance of complications), or use another structure that meets the aforementioned conditions. Obviously, surgical techniques have been eliminated that have proven inefficiency or limited duration of functionality.

2.2 Complications

Complications occurring in hydrocephalus surgery can occur at all levels of the location of the drainage tubular:

- upper pole - location of the proximal end of the tubules at the ventricular level

- middle segment - tubular dysfunctions

- lower pole - limitation of resorption capacity or complications at the level of the receiving structure.

The type of obstruction or over infection of the drainage tubular can occur at any level and tend to generalise.

The most common complications found are those of the distal segment, generally related to the inability of the receiving structure to take up the amount of excess cerebrospinal fluid, or systemic complications, which require the removal of the initial assembly and replacement with another surgical variant [9, 10].

3. Surgical techniques using the same receptor structures or derivatives

3.1 Ventriculoepiploic shunt

The involvement of the large epiplon in the resorptive processes of the peritoneum has long been known, but the qualities of this structure in the resorption of cerebrospinal fluid have not been tested. Intraperitoneal administration, or sub peritoneal injection of colourant solutions, led to the concentration of the substance in the ovoid structures of the large epiplon called "lactose spots" (Ranvier 1896). The microscopic observation of discontinuities in the mesothelial layer above the omental lactic patches (Muscatello) facilitates the contact with the vascular and lymphatic structures of the large epiplon, favouring the resorption phenomenon. Since the epiploic vessels are not affected by the process of atherosclerosis (regardless of the severity of this process at the systemic level), their resorptive power remains unchanged over time. If their calibre is generous enough, the distal catheter can be implanted directly into an epiploic vein [11].

The diverse cellularity of the large omentum (undifferentiated mesenchymal cells, macrophages, lymphocytes, adipocytes, etc.) facilitates the plasticity, resorptive power, and anti-infectious effect of this structure. The aforementioned qualities of this structure make it an "interesting" partner for draining the cerebrospinal fluid excess in hydrocephalus. The procedure can also be performed laparoscopically.

Technically, a gap is prepared between the sheets of the large epiplon, in which the distal end of the drainage tubing is located, and we fixed it with a non-obstructive wire to avoid the displacement from the insertion place [12, 13].

The advantages of the procedure are as follows:

- simple and risk-free surgical procedure

- the large epiplon is in direct contact with the anterior abdominal wall (the procedure is not laborious, and the surgical approach should not be wide)

- avoids contact, or significantly limits it, between the drainage tubing and the cerebrospinal fluid drained with the non-absorbing peritoneum, structurally and functionally modified by previous drainages at this level

- does not predispose to specific complications of the standard ventriculoperitoneal shunt (especially intestinal occlusions)

- can be relocated to other territories of the large epiplon if is need

- combines all the other advantages of ventriculoperitoneal shunt but avoiding direct contact of the cerebrospinal fluid and drainage tubing with the peritoneal serosa.

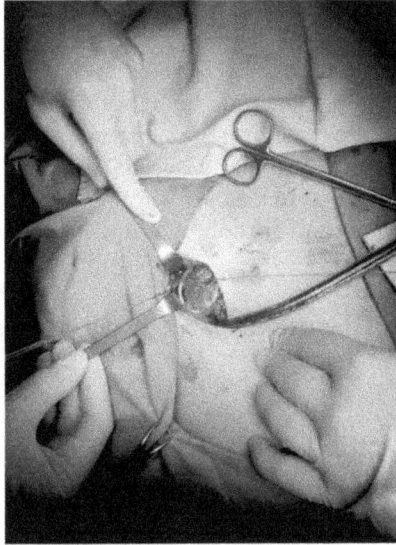

Figure 1.
Ventriculosubclavicular or ventriculocardiac shunt.

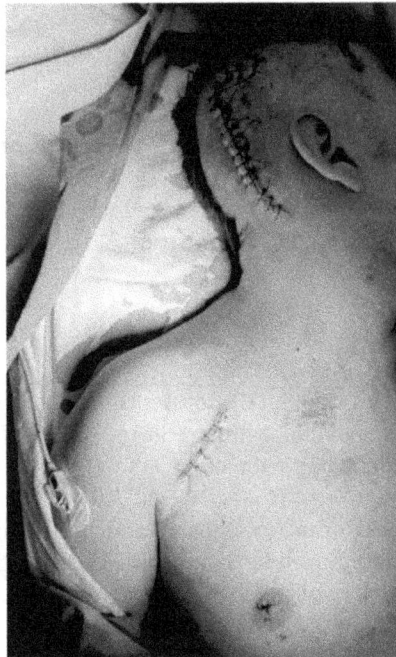

Figure 2.
Final view after the surgery is finish by right transcephalic approach (intraoperative view).

3.2 Ventriculosubclavicular or ventriculocardiac shunt by right transcephalic approach

It summarises all the advantages (but also records the disadvantages) of the standard (transjugular) ventriculocardiac shunt. The excess of cerebrospinal fluid is drained into the upper cavity/right heart system as well as into the ventriculocardiac shunt but uses another approach (angioaccess) when transjugular access is not possible or difficult to achieve.

The surgical procedure is simple to perform because of the anatomical proximity between the emerging catheter in the right lateral ventricle and the cephalic vein, which is discovered and catheterised into the right deltopectoral space. The progression of the distal end can be made up to the level of the right heart, and its position can be checked in the same way as in the case of the transjugular approach shunt. The procedure is technically simple and without major risks (**Figures 1** and **2**) [14].

4. Surgical techniques using other receptor structures for the excess of cerebrospinal fluid

Over time, surgical techniques have been tested using the pleural cavity, gallbladder, bladder, mastoid, ureters, etc., but the viability of these variants has been limited in time, or severe complications have been recorded that have compromised the method.

The vascular port remains an ideal receiver if the tubular path is not too long (predisposing to cuds or clogging), if the conditions of long-lasting and high sterility are met, and if the pressure gradients between the ventricular system and the receiving structure is enough. The venous structures meet such conditions, although they are" accused" of frequent thrombosis with early decomposition in conditions of insufficient blood flow or inadequate conduction of anticoagulant or antiplatelet therapy.

4.1 Transomphalic extraperitoneal ventriculoportal shunt

Is the first technique that does not drain the cerebrospinal fluid into the systemic circulation and uses functional hepatic circulation [15].

Advantages of the method:

- It is a physiological therapeutic solution

- The pressure gradient is enough (10–15 mm Hg in the ventricular system in the subject without hydrocephalus, compared to 5–10 mm Hg in the portal trunk in the subject without portal hypertension)

- Surgical technique does not raise any particular problems (identification and remediation of obliterated umbilical vein at the level of the round ligament of the liver generally can be made without difficulty)

- The transformation of the ventriculoperitoneal shunt into the transomphalic extraperitoneal ventriculoportal shunt can be achieved easily and without risks (the intermediate tubing can be easily detected paraumbilically right)

- Avoid the contact of tubes and cerebrospinal fluid with the abdominal visceral mass and anatomically and functionally modified peritoneum

- The liver can act as a barrier to germs, toxins, or immune complexes, limiting infectious complications or antibiotic regimens.

- Accumulates the advantages of classical drainage variants (ventriculoperitoneal and ventriculocardiac)

- Can be practiced by novo or as a viable therapeutic alternative in case of repetitive complications of the prescribed procedures.

4.2 Repermeabilisation of the umbilical vein

The umbilical vein approach can be made extraperitoneally or intraperitoneally. In the case of a ventriculoportal shunt, the extraperitoneal route is preferred, which presents multiple advantages, especially if there is a surgical history that altered the situation of the intestines and peritoneum itself (including multiple revisions of the ventriculoperitoneal shunt). The topographical proximity of the drainage tubing (if a ventriculoperitoneal shunt has previously worked) is an advantage that must be used. The juxtaumbilical segment of the round ligament of the liver at this level is extraperitoneal and can be identified in coalescence with the parietal peritoneum. Although it does not provide a generous visibility as in the intraperitoneal approach, in the thickness of the round ligament, the umbilical vein in various stages of obliteration can be easily identified, which is dissected and suspended on an anchor wire.

The approach to the vein can be done at this level or a little bit more proximal (closer to the liver) by creating a lateral slit. In the created gap is inserted a buttoned stiletto that progresses gently to the liver without major difficulties, up to the level of the venous estuary, where we encounter a resistance that must be overpassed gently. Crossing this obstacle confirms the penetration into the left portal frame. This can be checked by removing the catheterism stylus, which must confirm the reflux of portal blood. Portal manometry can be performed. The repermeabilisation of the vein should sometimes be supplemented by progressive Hegare dilation (4,6,8) until the required venous calibre is achieved for catheterisation. Progression of the distal end of the drainage system generally does not encounter difficulties, and at the end of the procedure, the catheter should be fixed with a safety wire.

Possible complications:

- Common complications associated with ventricular assembly or drainage tubing (elbows, disconnections, clogs)

- The overdrainage phenomenon

- Extra or subdural acute hematomas

- Ventricular slit syndrome

- Pneumocephalia

- Craniostenosis

- Portal vein thrombosis

Contraindications:

- Cirrhosis of the liver or other causes of portal hypertension

- Other liver diseases with a risk of liver failure

- Malignant haematological disorders

- Septic disorders of the intraperitoneal organs that are portal connected

- Digestive or extradigestive infectious diseases until to their therapeutic solution.

5. Conclusions

1. Ventriculoperitoneal shunt is the election method used in most of the cases of hydrocephalus (regardless of its aetiology), with good results, tolerance, and durability.

2. Ventriculocardiac shunt and ventriculocisternostomy (when indicated) are viable alternative options.

3. The indications for lumboperitoneal shunt and ventriculopleural shunt have progressively narrowed.

4. Ventriculoepiploic shunt, transomphalic extraperitoneal ventriculoportal shunt, and right cephalic ventriculosubclavicular/ventriculocaval/ventriculocardiac shunt represent backup solutions that can be used in case of repeated failure of the previously mentioned procedure.

Conflict of interest

The authors declare no conflict of interest.

Author details

Valentin Titus Grigorean[1,2*] and Alexandru Vlad Ciurea[3,4]

1 Department of General Surgery, University of Medicine and Pharmacy "Carol Davila", Bucharest, Romania

2 Emergency Clinical Hospital Bagdsar-Arseni, Bucharest, Romania

3 "Carol Davila" University of Medicine and Pharmacy, Bucharest, Romania

4 Sanador Clinical Center Hospital, Bucharest, Romania

*Address all correspondence to: valentin.grigorean@umfcd.ro

IntechOpen

References

[1] Isaacs AM, Riva-Cambrin J, Yavin D, Hockley A, Pringsheim TM, Jette N, et al. Age-specific global epidemiology of hydrocephalus: Systematic review, metanalysis and global birth surveillance. PLoS One. 2018;**13**:e0204926

[2] Bergsneider M, Miller C, Vespa PM, Hu X. Surgical management of adult hydrocephalus. Neurosurgery. 2008;**62**(Suppl):2

[3] Bothwell SW, Janigro D, Patabendige A. Cerebrospinal fluid dynamics and intracranial pressure elevation in neurological diseases. Fluids and Barriers of the CNS 2019. 2019;**16**(1):1-18

[4] Zanin L, Latour K, Suquet G, Panciani PP, Fiorindi A, Fontanella MM. Hydrocephalus and the first report of an external Ventriculostomy: The contributions of Fabrici d'Acquapendente in the Italian renaissance. World Neurosurgery. 2024;**188**:111-116

[5] Pillai S. Techniques and nuances in Ventriculoperitoneal shunt surgery. Neurology India. 2021;**69**:S457-S461. DOI: 10.4103/0028-3886.332261

[6] Bakhaidar M, Wilcox JT, Sinclair DS, Diaz RJ. Ventriculoatrial shunts: Review of technical aspects and complications. World Neurosurgery. 2022;**158**:158-164

[7] Yang TH, Chang CS, Sung WW, Liu JT. Lumboperitoneal shunt: A new modified surgical technique and a comparison of the complications with Ventriculoperitoneal shunt in a single Center. Medicina (B Aires). 2019;**55**:643

[8] Wong T, Gold J, Houser R, Herschman Y, Jani R, Goldstein I. Ventriculopleural shunt: Review of literature and novel ways to improve ventriculopleural shunt tolerance. Journal of the Neurological Sciences. 2021:**428**

[9] Merkler AE, Ch'ang J, Parker WE, Murthy SB, Kamel H. The rate of complications after Ventriculoperitoneal shunt surgery. World Neurosurgery. 2017;**98**:654-658

[10] Mottolese C, Beuriat PA, Szathmari A, Di Rocco F. Complications related to the treatment of hydrocephalus with Extrathecal cerebral spinal fluid shunts. Textbook of Pediatric Neurosurgery. 2019:1-33

[11] Grigorean VT, Popescu M, Sandu AM, Toader S. Ventriculo-epiplooic shunt, a new surgical technique for treatment of hydrocephalus. Journal of Experimental Medical and Surgical Research. 2010;**17**(1):55-63

[12] Grigorean VT, Sandu AM, Popescu M, Florian IS, Lupascu CD, Ursulescu CL. Our initial experience with ventriculo-epiplooic shunt in treatment of hydrocephalus in two centers. Neurologia i Neurochirurgia Polska. 2017;**51**:290-298

[13] Grigorean VT, Sandu AM. Alternative surgical therapy to standard treatment for hydrocephalus: Ventriculo-epiplooic shunt and ventriculoportal extraperitoneal transomphalic shunt. Proceedings of Romanian Academy, Series B. 2016;**18**:95-102

[14] Liţescu M, Cristian DA, Coman VE, Erchid A, Pleşea IE, Bordianu A, et al. Right Transcephalic Ventriculo-subclavian shunt in the surgical treatment of hydrocephalus—An original

procedure for drainage of cerebrospinal
fluid into the venous system. Journal of
Clinical Medicine. 2023;**12**:4919

[15] Grigorean VT, Sandu AM,
Popescu M, Strambu V. Ventriculoportal
shunt, a new Transomphalic
Extraperitoneal surgical technique in
treatment of hydrocephalus. Surgical
Innovation. 2017;**24**:223-232

www.ingramcontent.com/pod-product-compliance
Lightning Source LLC
Chambersburg PA
CBHW081336190326
41458CB00018B/6019